In this life here, we never can understand it until we fully live it with open eyes. I raised hell when I was young. I drank almost every day, and to find me sober was hard to do.

When I began to get sickly in my later years, I was in my locked room just as the sun was rising when a wanagi, a man dressed in the finest buckskin, came right through the door and spoke to me in the old way. The wanagi spirit spoke in the way spirits do and told me, "Purify yourself, purify your mind, and go up to find your way on the hill. They're waiting for you up there, Kola."

I was startled and sad. I didn't want this. I didn't want to be a Yuwipi. I ran from it until I couldn't anymore. It wasn't until they came after my children I gave in to it—two of my children died one night of a sudden and mysterious sickness. I went to the spirits and they told me they would keep coming after my family if I didn't go up on that hill, so I did. I prepared myself in the old way. I made two sacred pipes and took them up there with me four days and four nights with absolutely no food and no water.

It was on this hill my life changed forever and my eyes were opened to what life really is for the first time. The Coyote came first and he was singing a sacred song. He came really close then changed himself into a man painted red and blue. This man showed me how to make my Owanka and how to set it all up. Then the holy black-tailed deer came and he too was singing a sacred song, and he showed me the holy colors I would use in this Hocoka. Iktomi was next and he gave me good medicine and vowed to always be present to help me. The Wanbli Gleska flew over me and told me he would always bring the sick Wicozani, he said "Kola Wicozani Wakan Ota Akupi."

The ones to come last, one by one, were the stones and the ghosts of some of the past Yuwipi and they gave me good health and help like that, one by one. I was a new man. I was restored and I learned to walk a sacred road. There are always seventy-five spirits with me and some of them are always talking to me. Right here in this bad ear they speak to me. There is only one God, but there are many, many spirits on this earth. Open your eyes to your reality, for it is in front of you. When I pray in my Lakota way I pray in my words—we all need the same thing. We all need good health and help. Don't play with it. Don't play with your life. We need to help each other, to understand each other, to love each other."

—Agna Iyanka
Elmer Norbert Running
March 27th, 1993

Working with Grandpa

MY YEARS LIVING AND WORKING WITH THE OLDEST LIVING LAKOTA MEDICINE MAN, AND AFTERWARD

Karl Hamann

This book is memoir. It reflects the author's present recollections of experiences over time. Some names and characteristics have been changed, some events have been compressed, and some dialogue has been recreated.

Beaver's Pond Press is committed to turning interesting people into independent authors. In that spirit, we are proud to offer this book to our readers; however, the story, the experiences, and the words are the author's alone.

Softcover: ISBN 13: 978-1-64343-875-7
Hardcover: ISBN 13: 978-1-59298-805-1
Library of Congress Catalog Number: 2016918795
Printed in the United States of America
Hardcover edition first published in 2017.
First hardcover printing: 2017
Second softcover edition: 2020

24 23 22 21 20   5 4 3 2 1

Book design and typesetting by Tiffany Daniels

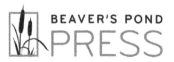

BEAVER'S POND
PRESS

Beaver's Pond Press
939 Seventh Street West
Saint Paul, MN 55102
(952) 829-8818
www.BeaversPondPress.com
To order, visit www.ItascaBooks.com
or call (800)-901-3480. Reseller discounts available.

THIS IS MY STORY OF THE TIME I WAS PRIVILEGED TO LIVE AND work with the last of the old-time Lakota *wicasa wakan*, or medicine men, Elmer Norbert Running. Although Grandpa was a twentieth-century Indian, he was the type of person I'd always wanted to meet, someone whose mind and heart were not set in the patterns of mainstream Western thought. For him, spiritual life, his own and that of his people, was the touchstone—not how well off he might be in relation to others, but how well he and those around him were in touch with Native tradition. This book is humbly dedicated to his life and work.

*Beware, white man, of playing
with the magic of the primitive. It
may be strong medicine. It may
kill you. Ye, sons and daughters,
foster children of the cities, if ye
would go to the wilderness in
search of your Mother, be careful
& circumspect, lest she lure you
into her secret places, whence ye
may not come back.*

—Jaime de Angulo, *The Lariat*

Contents

Preface

THIS IS A MEMOIR. ELMER RUNNING, THE MEDICINE MAN, whom I first met in 1997 and came to live with during most of 1999, was the most remarkable person I've ever met. He was the last of the old-timers, the medicine men, who grew up on the reservation of Rosebud, South Dakota, speaking Lakota with English a distant second. He was one of the humblest, most unassuming men around, and he lived, to the best of his ability, according to his peoples' ancient rules for such a man. For him—come hardship, come loss, come trials and betrayals—the people always came first. Not himself. As he always said, "Don't think about yourself. Just think about the people."

This story, the small part of it I experienced and can speak to, I've written in three parts. The first describes my year with him in 1999, on the Santee Reservation in Niobrara, Nebraska. The second tells about rejoining him late in 2000 at his original home on the Rosebud Reservation in South Dakota. The third part records a series of events that took place after his death in 2009. There is a gap of seven years, between 2001 and 2008, during which time I fell away before coming back.

Most of the book is a loosely chronological recounting of day-to-day events in the company of Elmer, who was often called

Grandpa, and others who participated in his ceremonies and sun dances—his family members, friends, and supporters. There are a few accounts of things that happened when the world and actions of the spirits intersected with our human sphere. In fact, that happened every month at his monthly *Iowampi* ceremonies and is only to be expected in any story about a medicine man.

I've indulged in a few rantings and diatribes when the situation of the Indian people seemed so outrageous I couldn't keep my mouth shut, figuratively speaking, but I don't claim to speak for any Indian people, and I don't set myself up as an expert on their customs and spiritual practices. This is just what I saw and heard and learned while I spent time with Grandpa.

Acknowledgments

I'D LIKE TO THANK ALL THE PEOPLE WHO HELPED ME TO WRITE this too-brief memoir of Elmer Norbert Running, or Agna Iyanka, as he was called in the language of his people.

Thanks for encouragement go to my old college roomie Chuck Dube, and to Elmer's brother, Al Running, who told me, "It's good you wrote something about my brother."

Thanks and *wopila tanka* to Michael Jagod for the photos and for keeping the lines of communication open.

To Gorgie Paulhamus for sharing her memories and insights.

Special thanks to Gwen Caldwell for believing in the old man when he told her, "The spirits, they said you're s'posed to come and take care of me."

To Dave Ross, for memories of shared work, play, and frustration—and his work recording and translating the old man's songs.

To Jason Kolbo, for all those hours at 3:00 a.m. and other times keeping fire and running the door.

And to all the sun dancers and supporters, for coming to pray.

Aho Mitakuye Oyasin.

PART I
Santee, 1999

CHAPTER I

Who Brought the Sage?

I FIRST MET ELMER NORBERT RUNNING IN 1997,
opagiing (offering a pipe to) him for his sun dance that year.
My soon-to-be ex-wife and I wanted to dance for the healing of
a little girl, the daughter of a Kiowa Vietnam veteran. She had
serious problems, including spina bifida and fluid on the brain.
By the time we returned to our home, these illnesses had been
healed. Her mother told us the white doctors at the VA hospital
couldn't believe it. I was impressed. So when our marriage fell
apart in 1999, I left Alabama and stayed with Grandma Darlene
Jackson in Minneapolis for a while. After a week or so, I was
together enough to wonder what was next, and she suggested I go
out to the home of Elmer and his wife, Patti, in Santee, Nebraska,
to stay and work and help out. It seemed like a good idea.

I arrived in late April or early May. It was still quite cold,
and I remember fetching in firewood for the little woodstove
in the living room for the first couple of weeks. There was also
Pete Mussel—who, if I recall, was Mdewakanton Dakota—
who was there as resident mechanic and to stay dry.

After a few weeks, the weather turned fair, and Pete and I
had been going out to the woods, cutting smaller ash trees for
uprights and stringers for the sun-dance arbor. During a wet

spell, I recall Elmer being grumpy about the rain: "Can't get out and do nothing!" Not much was done during the mornings. We sat around the TV, smoked, drank coffee—kind of all getting used to being together. By the time things dried out, it was almost time for Elmer and Patti to fly to Germany. He'd been asked to go and do a ceremony over there. For a bit, it was just me and Pete, but he soon left for a trip to the Twin Cities. So after about one month, I was on my own as a house sitter. By this time, I'd met Patti's son, Jamie, his daughter, and a few local folks.

The weather had been really very rainy. There was some question about whether or not Elmer and Patti could get out along the long gravel county road for their trip; parts of it were in danger of washing out. On the day of their departure, however, we had company. I got up to the old farmhouse, and there was a young man, a local Santee guy, and his small nephew. Elmer and Patti seemed to know him, so I didn't think any more of it, even though it meant they'd be there while I saw Elmer and Patti off.

Our two visitors left soon after I got back to the house. There was more rain that night, and earth-moving equipment was heading out our way, so the next morning, when this young man called me with a story about a parcel waiting for delivery to Elmer—which he'd be waiting with at the temporary road-head—I left to go get it.

When I arrived at the point where the road crew had closed the road, no one was there. He used my absence to get in along the other approach and steal Elmer's portable generator. When I called him to see what happened, he had some confusing story about the package being already at the post office, and sorry for the mix-up. The theft wasn't detected until Elmer and Patti got back, some ten days later. The first evening, Elmer did the rounds of the property. "Gonna look around," he said as he left. He was back soon, and angry. "Generator's gone!" Patti got after me a little bit, but we eventually figured out what had happened. Jamie called this guy up and chewed him out for deceiving me—and, of course, for the theft.

We were sure it was him; he had a reputation on the rez for that kind of thing. And months later, as the time for the sun dance got closer, he came back because he wanted to dance that year. The afternoon he showed up, he was out behind the house by the workshop shed, waiting for Elmer. I was still kind of mad at him for ripping off the old man and for making me look bad, so I headed out there with a grim look on. When he saw me, he got scared and ducked behind a big cable spool Elmer used as a worktable. I decided then, or rather I remembered, it was against tradition to bring anger or violence around a *wicasa wakan*. So I didn't even approach him.

A while later, on my way back inside, I saw this fellow and Elmer sitting out back there, and Elmer was holding this man's *canunpa* (or sacred pipe), pointing to it and obviously explaining something to him.

In that moment, I realized that although he'd been upset by the loss of his equipment, Elmer couldn't, wouldn't, hold it against this youngster. He would help him, instruct him, and not mind it any more than if a dog lifted his leg against his lodgepole, to use an old expression. That's when I began to understand what it meant to be a man called by the spirits for his people—and how humbling it was to see.

Years later, I fell away for a long time, but the spirits called me back in 2008, and I am so glad I listened. I'll never forget that year I got to spend and work with Elmer, when I was beginning to learn the things I should do before I sun danced, going to his monthly ceremony, helping with sweat, and all the rest. How I miss him now and look forward to seeing him when I cross over! As I write this, in the spring of 2012, I'm almost physically sick with worry over the Mother Earth, how badly she's been used. Every year we have fewer and fewer men like Grandpa, and every year we need them more and more. Remember his words, you sun dancers and others: "Don't think about yourself. Just think about the people."

Before the incident with the generator, though, there was the business with the sage. That was in early May, and it was still cold. A little time had passed since the last monthly ceremony, and the sweat lodges hadn't been cleaned out. The coming weekend, there was a special doctoring ceremony to be held for some folks, and we were out of sage for the sweat. I was itching for something to do, so Elmer had me use a wheelbarrow to clean out the rocks. A thin mist, almost sleet, was falling. I began gathering the rocks, putting them into the wheelbarrow, and wheeling them between the ceremony house and the woods, out to the edge of a little bank, where they were dumped. Just in front and to the left of the ceremony house, a pine tree was growing, and the carpet of dead needles beneath the boughs was dry. I went back for a second load of rocks, using my gloved hands to scrape up the smaller pieces. Out to the dump again, but as I passed the pine, lo and behold, there on the dry needles was a large bundle of dried sage! It couldn't have been there on my first trip, and no one else was around outside. Everyone was inside, keeping out of the weather. I picked up the sage, wondering. Then I hung it up inside the changing shed next to the sweat lodges.

After I finished cleaning up, I put away the wheelbarrow and went inside. I took off my boots, came into the living room, sat down, and said, "Elmer, I found a bundle of sage under the pine by the ceremony house. It wasn't there before."

He looked a little surprised for a moment, then smiled and just said, "Somebody must've brought it." And that was all.

As the days passed into spring, while Elmer and Patti were in Germany, Pete and I (before he left for a brief trip) spent our time cutting crutches and stringers of ash for the sun-dance arbor. Pete had told me early on that he wasn't a sun dancer, just an ordinary Indian who was trying to stay sober.

We also did a little mowing, since the grass around the farmhouse was just beginning to get long. One morning, trying to start a cold push mower, Pete mentioned something so basic to the mechanics of mowers that I had to say, "Pete, I know about that!"

His response was, "Ah, but you wouldn't believe some of the people we get here who want to help out and don't know what they're doin'! Like one guy last year—he took that other mower and was doing the yard and ran it over something, hard, bent the shaft, and just put it away without saying nothin'! Then there was the guy who said he'd get me some tools, a whole set of sockets and drivers, half inch, three-quarters, so I could do some real work on the vehicles here. He left, came back, and all he brought was this little dinky set of one-fourth inch, with one little ratchet."

"Wow," was all I could say in response. This kind of talk put me on my guard; I felt I'd have to do good work so I wouldn't get lumped in with the other white guys who came to help and turned out to be more of a hindrance.

Pete left for a short trip, and after about a week or so on my own, Elmer and Patti got back. After the incident with the generator settled down, people from the Santee community and farther afield would stop by for a visit. Among them was Patti's son, Jamie, and his little daughter, about four or five years old, whose name escapes me. And one evening, while Elmer had been working at his pipe carving in his little shop in a small room just off the living room, a young man, obviously a full blood, came in to offer a pipe to him. Indians, at least the traditional ones, aren't much for kneeling to anybody. But this guy waited until Elmer came out and sat down in his chair, then got down on his knees to *opagi*. It seemed everyone I met had the greatest respect for the man—except for the one closest to him, and his family.

We got a call, a week or so after this, to have Elmer come and bless a new drum for use by a new group of singers in Sioux Falls, South Dakota. After a long drive, we arrived at the Catholic church, in whose basement community room the ceremony was to take place. As we waited, I noticed from the backseat of the Aerostar a priest arriving and entering the building. "There's Father," I said. I was about to launch into a speech about how I'd been raised Lutheran and been confirmed but how I had never experienced anything like the power of ceremony or seen dramatic healings and recoveries as a result of Christian prayer, when Elmer did something he almost never did. He cut me off before I could get started and told me that white people were always telling him how they'd been raised Christian but had never experienced the power of his ceremony in a Christian service or seen such dramatic healings. "That's what they tell me," he finished, kind of glaring at me.

I stayed pretty quiet the rest of that day. I got even quieter when, during his address to the members and families of the new drum group, he talked about how life had been so good for his people before the coming of the whites, the *wasicus*. "Then they took it away from us, everything." It's one thing to read about it in the history books, but it's a whole lot different when you're the only non-Indian in a room full of them. I felt my country's evil legacy of attempted genocide bearing down on me in a way I'd never felt before, and I hated it.

When I was younger, I had absorbed the antiestablishment values of the youth of the late 1960s and early 1970s, and I'm here to say America likes to believe itself to be one thing, the land of the free and the home of the brave, but after having lived on the rez and learning how Leonard Peltier, and the members of American Indian Movement (AIM), and the occupiers of Wounded Knee have been treated—not to mention the FBI's firebombing of the home of activist John Trudell, resulting in the deaths of his wife and some of their children, and the ongoing war of genocide—I have to say that, despite the many privileges and freedoms offered to you if you are the right color and gender, this country is nothing more than a lying, racist, murdering imperium. I was raised to love my country, but after the murders of Dr. Martin Luther King Jr., the Kennedys, Anna Mae Aquash, Fred Hampton, Martha Honey, and Karen Silkwood to name but a few, it's obvious to me that when the Yippies called America schizophrenic, they were right on the money. White people, and many of the blacks too, are mostly all crazy. They destroy life, and the foundation of life, the sacred Mother Earth, for a few dollars, and they think this makes them responsible providers for their families, and big men and women. But can someone tell me why the buffalo were all but wiped out and why the illegal liquor stores on the borders of the Oglala reservation remain open? If it doesn't boil down to profiting from genocide, I'd like to hear it.

Chapter 2

A Medicine Man's Funeral

THE NEXT INSTANCE OF ELMER, PATTI, AND ME GOING ON A trip together was to attend the funeral—though not the burial—of a well-known medicine man who had lived with his family a short way north of the Missouri River in South Dakota. I seem to recall his name as Steve Red Buffalo, though I can't be sure. We left in the late afternoon and arrived in the early evening. We'd been stopped by the South Dakota state patrol just after we crossed the river, and Patti had gotten a ticket for not wearing her safety belt. She'd filled me in on the way up. It seems this man had been working on one of his vehicles a few days previously. He'd gotten it running and taken it out for a test drive. While motoring along at a moderate speed, not far from his home, he had somehow lost control on a patch of gravel, had been thrown clear, and was killed instantly. Alcohol and drugs weren't involved. I heard that at least one of the medicine man's teenage daughters had failed to comport herself in the manner proper to the child of a *wicasa wakan*, and her father's uncanny demise had been the result. Seems the spirits really hadn't liked how she'd been carrying on.

When we arrived, quite a few people were in attendance.
A large tipi had been set up in the front yard of the house, and
the sky was clear, the air was dry, and no wind blew. It was just
before sundown when the memorial ceremony began. A drum
group began a loud, strong beat, then the voices of the singers
chanting and wailing, one single high voice at first with the rest
taking up and repeating it. I remember that about this time, the
deceased's wife, a tall, matronly woman, came over to greet us,
flung her arms around Patti, and cried, "Oh, Patti! What am I
gonna do?" It was hard to watch, but Patti was steady and began
to offer some words of comfort.

Then, as people began to file into the tipi, where the body
was lying in full ceremonial regalia, and where the drum was, the
daughter arrived. Surrounded by women who were probably her
aunts and other close relatives, she came weeping uncontrollably.
Being borne up by her supporters as much as by her own efforts,
she screamed out, "I want my dad!"

I had to turn away. I took a place in line, went in and took
part in the visitation, and came out again. I was so moved, I took
a bill out of my wallet and asked Patti to tell the widow I wanted
to give it to her. Patti introduced me, saying, "This is Karl. He's
staying with us, and he'd like to give you this little bit of money."
If Elmer made any prayers, or officiated in any other way, I
didn't see.

I recall other events that took place early on, such as the first
time Elmer left me to do a job on my own. A local guy about my
own age, called Nico, had come in and was visiting just after
someone else had dropped off a big load of firewood. Elmer and
Nico and I had helped pitch it off the truck, then Elmer told me
to stack it on the pile "in a nice way" so the fire keepers wouldn't
have to wrestle it out.

I repeated the instruction to Nico, who said, "If that's what
he said, that's what he meant." So that's what I did. Stacked it

all nice and neat so the ends wouldn't bind on each other. That weekend, it rained, and we were trying to get the fire started for the sweat before the monthly ceremony. It was important we get started more or less on time since there was a party in attendance, one of whom had requested a doctoring. But it was no-go—even with the inner bark of the cottonwood. Finally, Elmer looked up and told me, "Karl, go get that tractor oil. Pour it on." He meant a jug of hydraulic fluid over by the toolshed. I poured it on the kindling underneath the cradle of logs that formed the base of the coneshaped stack of wood and stones, and that got it going once we put a match to it! We had a hot sweat that evening, if I remember right, and a good ceremony. I remember, too, just before I'd unscrew the lightbulb, to ensure total darkness in the ceremony house so the spirits could come in, the door would be locked. I was told that this was to make sure some rambunctious spirit wouldn't fling it open and let in light from the security lamp on the power pole or moonlight. Apparently, this had happened once before, and Elmer was determined to be careful.

Elmer and Patti had three dogs living with them who had all just sort of showed up and stayed on at various times. There was Waziya, the big female shepherd mix, definitely the alpha female. Tegi was a little black pit bull–mongrel male. The third was a smaller yellow short-hair female whose name escapes me. Waziya was very friendly, the yellow one was a slinking cur, and Tegi had a definite attitude. As Nico put it, "He thinks he's king shit."

The other thing about Tegi was that anytime someone turned down the dirt track from the gravel county road toward the yard, he'd stand and howl. Every time, without fail. If the mail truck stopped at the mailbox, or if a vehicle drove past, there'd be no response. This is significant because of what happened during sweat, before the second-to-last monthly ceremony. It would have been on the night of the new moon in June that year, since that was always ceremony time. In addition to a few sun dancers and attendees who were local regulars, Jamie, Nico, and a white guy from Milwaukee named Dave Ross—who'd been coming to Elmer's for years and had produced a digital recording and booklet with translations of Elmer's ceremony and sun-dance songs—there was a party in from out of state, whose members were there for another doctoring. So I recall that spirits were high that Saturday afternoon. Dave and I were tending to the fire, while Jamie and Nico were listening to a new powwow CD—I think it was the Whitefish Bay Singers. I recall they were listening to one track where one of the singers had an incredibly high falsetto. In Indian singing, the higher the male lead voice can get, the better, at least in Northern style. Kind of like white blues guys in the 1970s, but coming from a much older tradition. Anyway, this guy was higher than anyone I'd ever heard, and Jamie, who was a singer himself, said, "Oooh! He's got to stop doing that! I don't like that!" And Tegi made us all laugh by lying down in the middle of the lane in the yard, with his front paws crossed, and barking as if in rebuke of the situation generally. Just a reminder of who he thought was who around here.

A few hours later, just as it was getting dark, we all went in to sweat. I say *we*, but I was the man on the door that night, which meant I stayed outside and brought the rocks with a pitchfork, fed the grandfathers in, passed in the bucket of water, took it out when empty, and handed in Elmer's *canunpa* during the third round. There was also the opening of the door, a flap of canvas, after each round, when I heard the cry of *"Mitakuye Oyasin!"* from those within. Everything was going as usual; Patti was over in the women's lodge, leading the women who'd come in with the doctoring party. I was on both doors, so I was pretty busy. The women finished first and headed over to the changing shed, just north of the men's lodge. By now, it was full dark. The men were on their last round, when suddenly Tegi set up a howl fit to wake the dead. But there was no one coming down the lane. At almost the same time, the men's song was cut short, and one of the party thrust the flap open from the inside, which you're not supposed to do. I walked up as the men were coming out, and the guy who was there to be doctored said, "You'd better check on the old man. He's pretty sick." I poked my head in, and Elmer was sitting in his usual spot, to the left of the entrance, but all slumped over and not saying anything. So I ran and got Patti, and she came out and spoke to him. I recall overhearing him saying, "That's it."

Patti responded, "No, come on. Get up. We'll help get you out of there."

So she called to Dave and me, and we helped Elmer over to one of the picnic tables that sat between the ceremony house and the old farmhouse and got him sat down with a dry towel over him. Then she had Dave get a flat-bottomed spade and fill it with embers from the fire, while I was told to get a big chunk of dried mushroom that was sitting as a door prop on the floor of Elmer's workroom. I brought it out, we put it on the coals in the spade, and when it was smoldering good, giving off a heavy, weird-smelling smoke, she told me to smudge Elmer, the sweat lodges, the changing house, inside the house itself, and all present. Turns out, that mushroom was *wanagi pejuta*, ghost medicine. An evil spirit had come into the sweat lodge and attacked Elmer. That was the arrival Tegi's howl had announced. After he was smudged off with it, Elmer rallied considerably and seemed to come back to himself, although still kind of shook up.

He told us, "That spirit came right into the sweat! He said, 'I'm gonna take your power, and alla your songs.' He was a little one."

"Did he say his name?" I asked. And Elmer looked at me kinda funny and just said, "Shorty."

I honestly can't recall if we went through with the doctoring ceremony that night or if we went for it the following evening.

By this time, it must have been getting on toward late June. I
remember taking a trip back to the Twin Cities to visit the Ojibwa
elder, Darlene Jackson, who'd suggested I go out to Santee and
help Elmer. When I got there, there were young people sprawled
all over her living room floor, asleep. Dar, or "Bozhoo," as she
liked to be called, told me they were protesters who were taking
a break from an encampment set up to protect two huge old oak
trees. These had been identified as Dakota burial trees, where
the old ones had put the bodies of their departed. They were
scheduled to be cut down to make way for a new high-speed light
commuter rail line.

I remember going to a hearing in the county courthouse
and listening to an Indian lawyer argue for their preservation.
He made some remarks in an opening statement about how the
process of putting all the tribes east of the Mississippi into Indian
Country, or Oklahoma, as like "one big concentration camp." You
could sense the hostility from the county officials. I remember
the police on duty at the hearing were very overbearing and
insolent. When I went out for a smoke, one lady cop told me
that if I exited the hearing, I wouldn't be allowed back in. Later,
during a brief recess, I went out with several of the others, and,
on my way back inside, I looked her right in the eye, and she
couldn't face me.

When I was back for another visit to Dar, later on in the fall,
she showed me a videotape of the police forcibly dismantling the
camp and just throwing the contents into a van; there was no
respect for any possessions of the protestors. Later still, the trees
were cut and the rail line built. It reminds me of what the British
singer Ian Hunter of Mott the Hoople said of this country on
tour when he observed a colonial-era building, which had been a
historical site, scheduled for demolition: "Cute how they destroy
what culture they have." But having mostly devoured Native
rights, culture, and the land base in the first four hundred years

of its existence, America now seems bent not only on raping away what little is left but also consuming itself.

On the way back to Santee, I stopped at a little hardware store in a small town in western Minnesota that had cans of sale paint out front. I got five or six gallons of white, red, black, blue, yellow, and green. Elmer and Patti were on the road again, doing ceremonies for folks elsewhere, and it was just Pete and me back at the homestead. The sun-dance arbor was rebuilt, but many of the crutches—the forked uprights—weren't stripped of their bark or painted. I had to ask Pete if I could use Elmer's favorite short axe, a nice Estwing, that was stashed in the pickup. He teased me a little about using the chief's axe but said OK. So as the weather turned hot, I was in the shade of the cottonwoods, stripping off bark and repainting both the old and new crutches of the arbor. Dave had returned to Wisconsin, but one or two other sun dancers showed up to lend a hand.

One morning about Midsummer Day, I was up later than usual, working on something or other, and Elmer and I sat down together at the picnic table for a break and a smoke. He said nothing at first, then told me he'd just seen a spirit woman. He'd been down looking over the sun-dance grounds, said this figure had just appeared to him as an Indian woman dressed in a white buckskin dress and simply looked at him. I asked him if she'd said anything, and he told me no. Looking back on it thirteen years later, I'd say he seemed a little perturbed by it. I'm glad I began writing these memoirs of my time with him at the same seasons of the year as the experience itself. Somehow the consonance of the season makes it easier to remember. About this time, I recall that I either bought or traded the old man for a little camper he had sitting out back. My own homemade camper, a 1995 Ford E350 high-cube moving van I'd converted, was perfectly adequate to my needs, but I felt I was going to be staying around for a while. There was certainly nowhere else I wanted to be.

It was at about this time, when the evenings were starting to get long, that Elmer's son Gilli showed up for a visit. This was the first of Elmer's many children that I'd meet, and I didn't take to him in a big way. During my first two years, I'd heard that after Elmer's first wife had passed away, they'd nearly all started drinking—and stealing from their father to pay for it. Even things used in ceremony, like the painted buffalo skulls in front of the sweat lodges. This, I'd been told, was the reason Elmer was living in Santee in Nebraska, instead of where he was from, Ironwood on the Rosebud rez in South Dakota. To be quite candid, Gilli, with his nervous and undisguised expression of calculation, put me in mind of a vulture circling around waiting for something to die. I regret to say I've never had any reason to revise that first impression. Gilli didn't stay long, and it wasn't long afterward that Elmer had a fall from his tractor. I'd been down with him at the parking area, helping him mow, and I was right behind the tractor when he stopped the engine and got up to get down. I managed to catch him and stop the fall. "Good thing you was right there!" he said, and we made our way up to the house for lunch. This wasn't to be the last time that I was to catch the old man after he'd been made ill, or at least unsteady, by the presence of one of his offspring who wasn't walking in a good way, as the saying goes. Like the medicine man whose funeral we'd attended, the spirits would take it out on Elmer for the transgressions of his kids and sun dancers. I don't know why they do this. It must have to do with the kinship structures and obligations of tribal life. That's as much as I can guess.

But getting back to current events, the roof of my new camper had water stains in the ceiling. Obviously the roof leaked, and when I brought this to Elmer's attention, he told me, "Just throw some tobacco up there. That'll stop that leakin'."

So I kept the camper for the time being, but as things turned out, I ended up moving it, along with everything else, to the new house. But it was about this time, early on in July, that the four riders showed up. Four Indian men on horseback, riding cross-country to raise awareness of Native traditions and treaty rights. The subject of termination of all treaty obligations had come up in Congress, and there was even a bill to the same end, sponsored by some wretched junior Republican yahoo. I wish I could recall the riders' names, but I only remember that they stayed a couple of days, slept in the ceremony house, which was standard procedure for overnight guests, and a little bit of happenstance and conversation while they were with us. With four guests, plus Pete and myself in the little farmhouse, seating space in the living room was at a premium. One time, I took a seat recently vacated by the leader. When he came back in from the kitchen and saw me there, he jokingly pulled out a knife and pretended to threaten me with it, unless I got out! So I got right up, just playing along. Everyone was laughing, and Elmer got up out of his easy chair in the corner and went to work in his little shop, first saying, "That's the chief's chair. You gonna sit in that, you gonna have a hard time!"

And he was right! Of all the broken-springed, blanket-padded, uncomfortable seats I've ever taken, that one was the worst. It was a backbreaker. His words about a chief's seat being hard meant more than just this, I knew, but the reality was more than enough. Someone who serves the people and puts himself behind them and under the spirits has it pretty rough. Once in ceremony, I remember him telling us about people who wanted to be medicine men: "You get to be medicine man, you gonna pay a big pay."

As to the conversation in the living room, the leader of the band of riders held forth for a while, talking of how the first white people had come to be called *wasicu*—a sort of pun-

ning reference to the north wind, *waziya*, whose color is white.
But it also refers to a sort of mischievous imp spirit thought to
inhabit the grounds where many buffalo were butchered. If any
choice cuts were found to be missing, it was said the *wasicu* had
taken them. Hence, the fat-takers. I've also heard that when the
vast herd of buffalo were first sighted, the scout would report,
"Wasicu," meaning in this instance, "beyond counting." I don't
know which is right. He also spoke of how, if one were to take
the life of another wrongfully, one's spirit might be pursued by
that death down through seven generations.

The only other thing I remember from the time of their visit
is that I walked down to the camping area next to the sun-dance
grounds just to look at the horses. They had picketed them on
long leads, and one of the mounts had managed to tangle itself
so badly it was practically lashed up against one of the big cottonwoods. There was just enough slack for me to approach and,
speaking soothingly, get it loose.

I may have confused the timing of the riders' visit. It was
most likely sometime in August, after a sun dance. I know that
because I recall I went back to Omaha for a family visit after a
sun dance, and after the flood, and after Patti had gotten us the
new place. On my way south, I distinctly remember passing the
riders, who had left just that morning.

Pete Mussel, our mechanic, decided about three weeks before
the sun dance that he'd had enough of sobriety for a while. I gave
him a ride to some little town he knew, and the next evening, he
called up, drunk as a boiled owl and wanting to talk to Patti's
granddaughter, whom I'd been minding all afternoon. The next
day was noteworthy because I got my first Lakota teasing. We
were in the little living room, I had my towels and a change of
clothes, ready for a shower, but somehow I was just dithering,
and Patti and Elmer were getting impatient. So I went in and
showered, and it seemed to be no big deal—until the next time,

a day or so later, when Elmer commented, "You got your buddy with you?"

"Huh?" I replied, not getting it at all.

"Your porcupine buddy."

"Oh! Him!" I yelped, mightily embarrassed because what Elmer had just said to me in a Lakota idiom was, "You smell."

Elmer and I were busy every day during the last few weeks before the sun dance. Pete was still away, and Dave Ross hadn't gotten back yet. Jamie and Nico were around some, but they both had jobs in town. It used to be that some folks would come early to help get things ready, but this year there was less of this. "Them Indians gettin' smart," Elmer would say, grinning. "They wait 'til everything, it's ready, then show up!"

One bunch had come in while I'd been away and had dropped off an outhouse they said they'd spent five hundred dollars on. Apart from a few stray guys, a young Lakota man, and a guy from Germany who helped Nico and I stack firewood, there weren't too many, though.

There were a lot of folks who came in at various times, however, to be put up on the hill, for *hanblechiya*, or "lamenting," as it's known in Lakota, or "vision quest." One party of such people pulled into the yard one Friday afternoon and made the mistake of leaving the car windows rolled down. I was taking a break after the day's work when I saw, quick as a wink, the little yellow dog jump into the car through the open window, grab a bag of some kind of snacks, jump out again, and run off! I also remember being alone down by the grounds when a spotted fawn shot past me, almost brushing my leg. A moment later, Tegi and Waziya shot through in hot pursuit. They got it; I stumbled upon the carcass the next day.

According to tradition, being the woman of the house, Patti was supposed to feed and look after the dogs. About this time, I remember her going outside one morning with a can of scraps that had been left so long the top was bright blue with mold. Tegi backed up a step with a look of shock. Patti was getting strange, and more than a little mean. She'd gotten after me for being asleep the night the generator was stolen, but I'd gone back in and defended myself, and she'd admitted that I did, in fact, have to sleep sometimes. I mentioned it to Elmer afterward, sitting out on one of the sweat-lodge benches, and he'd laughed.

"What's so funny?" I asked, but he just grinned.

About this time, we had a little tornado scare one evening when the warnings were on TV. A sudden eerie stillness fell over the sky, and the weird green clouds rolled in, but it went by us. Later on, Patti remarked how one never heard of a tornado striking an Indian reservation. That made me sit up and realize she was right. Except once, up in a smaller rez in South Dakota, a few years previously, it had happened. "They didn't have no medicine man up there," said Elmer.

CHAPTER 3

The Great Flood

AFTER THIS, THE RAINS BEGAN TO COME IN HARD. ONE MORN-
ing, Elmer and I had to go down to the parking area north of
the arbor with our chainsaws, because a big old cottonwood had
come down in the soft earth. Unfortunately, the trunk was up off
the ground some ten feet at the crown. The tree was being supported by one of its larger limbs, the end of which had snapped
off and been driven into the soil. A timberman's nightmare. Once
the support was cut through, there was no way to predict how
the trunk would fall. Well, we set to work limbing the crown
first, then went at the support. I knew Elmer was a trifle deaf,
as well as having one glass eye, so when the trunk began to shift
and groan, I said something to him.

Man, he could still move pretty fast for a seventy-eight-year-
old who'd suffered a stroke late in the winter! I recalled what
Patti had told me soon after I'd arrived. After he'd suffered the
stroke and been to the hospital, she'd called a medicine man out
in Pine Ridge, Rick Two Dogs, and requested a long-distance doctoring. Elmer was partly paralyzed on one side and had said to
her, "The people are gonna kill me." Patti said she'd known just
what he'd meant—that some of his sun dancers and ceremony-go-
ers had either been drinking or otherwise misbehaving, and he

had to pay for it. But the long-distance doctoring took. He'd completely recovered from the paralysis in just a few weeks, which is very unusual in a man that age. But both of us got out of the way as the big trunk came down. We spent the rest of the morning cutting it up into firewood and hauling it back into the old garage that was also the woodshed.

It was about this time that Dave Ross got back from his job, saying he'd be around to help out until sun dance. With Pete still gone, it was good to have another pair of hands around, especially since they belonged to such a cheerful and willing guy. He was there to stay with Elmer while Nico and I made a run into Minneapolis to visit Grandma Darlene, who guided us to a vast army surplus store where we were to buy a huge, two-story canvas tent for use as a cookshack or some such. I forget whose idea it was, but the trip with Nico was, well, a trip. He almost never shut up, his trailer had no working taillights, and he brought along his young son. First, just after sundown, after we'd been on the road for a couple of hours, we stopped at a convenience store for gas, duct tape, two red bandannas, and two small flashlights. With batteries and five minutes' work, we had two fake-out taillights. Then we stopped at a little town on the Nebraska–South Dakota border for dinner and a rest stop, and he wanted to go into a titty bar, leaving his boy asleep in the backseat of his pickup. I wasn't up for the idea at all, and since somehow it had gotten to be my run, I had the say. I recall Dave and Elmer had each pitched in about a hundred bucks, with me to make up the difference.

We got to Bozhoo's all right, went to the store, and watched while a tall forklift dumped this huge folded pile of canvas into the trailer. We were gone three or four days, and when we got back, Dave was in town. Nico dropped the trailer down at the bottom of the sun-dance grounds, by the old cookshack, and took his boy home. I went off to look for Elmer. I think it was the first time he greeted me with the traditional Lakota greeting between two males: *"Hau-hau-hau!* Sun dance gettin' really close now!" He seemed in high spirits as we loaded a fridge, or "Frigidaire," as he invariably called it, onto the back of his pickup and took it down to the old cookshack.

A lot of people came to Elmer's sun dance in Santee: Indians from his old outfit in Ironwood in Rosebud, where he'd started, folks from Santee, the Isanti Dakota, a few Poncas, part of whose reservation had been ceded by the government to the Isanti after the troubles in 1862, whites from all over, plus, every year the Germans.

The days were getting to be really hot. A new fellow from Saint Paul, who also knew Darlene, showed us one afternoon that the heat index for northern Nebraska was closer to what was usually found in the tropics. This was due in part to all the rain we were getting. After Elmer and I had set the fridge on a pallet to keep the motor dry and plugged it in, he asked me if I thought we should unplug it, it being so hot. I answered, "No, it should be OK," thinking it was almost evening.

The next day we went back to unload some hundred-pound propane tanks for the cookstove, and the motor had burned overnight, completely fried. "I guess we shoulda unplugged it," I mumbled.

"That's the Frigidaire of the people!" Elmer replied. I didn't quite get him.

We set up a couple of tall crutches the next night, for setting up the big canvas tent, but it was too much. Without a full crew, there was no way to deal with all that bulky weight.

Elmer, Dave, and I had discussed plans for mowing the entire grounds once more. The grass was getting too high with all the rain. That night, one week before the beginning of purification, lying in my bunk in my homemade camper, I was awakened by the rain coming down so fast and hard I thought it'd beat a hole in the roof. The thunder was practically continuous; the interior was lit by incessant lightning. Took me a long time to get back to sleep, and when I awoke the next morning, it was to find several feet of swiftly flowing water almost into the edge of the backyard where I was parked.

All the recent deluge had carried years' worth of bankside flotsam downstream to some narrows and formed a dam. All the low-lying ground on the west side of Beaver Creek was under several feet of water, even extending upstream from Elmer's property. The old farmhouse, outbuildings, and sweat lodges were on high ground, but the land fell away gently to the north, where the sun-dance arbor, parking and camping areas, and the cookshack were. Fortunately, the dam itself had been swept away before the waters rose as high as the backyard. But the five-hundred-dollar outhouse was gone, as well as two of the other four we'd put in place. The propane tanks had been carried into the woods behind the cookshack, and there was no more need to mow; a solid inch of silt had been deposited evenly over the flooded area!

Dave Ross was in a motel in Niobrara that night. A young NDN man sent by the tribe came out to check on Elmer and Patti. He arrived about the same time I finished my coffee, and Elmer came outside. The water had by now receded to where we could walk down to where the road jogged in toward the creek, but between there and the grounds was a swiftly flowing channel about fourteen feet wide and eight inches deep. I'd finished my visit to the outhouse and caught up to them and stood there watching as this fellow carefully forded Elmer across, keeping himself upstream. Elmer was really quiet on the trek back up to the house, only exchanging a few words of Lakota/Dakota with the young man.

I think it was that morning I got spider-bit in the outhouse. There was nothing to be done until the water subsided, and I recall a day about then when we were all spending the afternoon in the living room and I was out of it—achy, mildly feverish, and all my joints hurt. "It's all this rain," I told myself, but that night I discovered a huge, fluid-filled blister on the bottom of my right (nether) cheek, which of course I could only feel. Classic brown recluse venom effect, but I thought it strange, since one of Elmer's principal helping spirits was the spider, or Iktomi. But no stranger than a medicine man's dance arbor getting flooded!

Dave got there just as we all reached the backyard, and I filled him in on the news. He said the road between Elmer's and the highway was almost impassable due to land slippage. When Elmer went back inside and sat down with his inseparable cigarette and cup of coffee, he was angry and downcast. "That's it! No sun dance this year!"

"Oh, no, just wait. There's still a week to go," Patti replied.

Dave and I got up and left them to it. Outside, I mentioned how quiet Elmer had been on the way back from viewing the grounds.

"I think he was in shock!" Dave said, and he was right. There was nothing anyone could do, so Dave drove into town after asking Patti if he were to buy some chicken, would she fry 'em? She agreed, so we had a nice dinner that night to cheer us up.

Thankfully, there was no more rain. As the land dried out over the next several days, we found and reset the three remaining outhouses and set up the cookshack—and Elmer began trying to regrade the road with his tractor.

I guess a description of the house and grounds would be helpful here. After turning south off the state highway that leads into Niobrara, one traveled south for five or six miles, sometimes at the top, but mostly below the ridge of a bluff that faced east. There were several widely spaced farms and houses along the road, with their driveways and neatly lettered mailboxes. At the base ran a little stream, a continuation of the Beaver Creek, which ran in back of Elmer's, which was on the opposite side. At one or two points there were constant washout problems due to outflow from springs. Patti had told me that when the engineers were siting the road, the farmers had told them where the springs were, but they were ignored. After it rained, there were always some graders and gravel dumpers at work.

I recall that one wet day before the flood, Patti and I were on a half-day road trip to some little town thirty miles away to see about buying a little camper. "Look at those *heyokas*!" she exclaimed, referring to the huge storm clouds building in from the west. She told me about the old-timers warning the government surveyors, and I seem to recall that where the road joined the highway, there was water flowing through a culvert below, but out at Elmer's it was farther east. The land leveled out there, with the line of hills to the west, some flat fields, the road, Elmer's outfit, and the creek about a half mile down on lower ground. Beaver Creek meandered, of course, so that the land between it and the road widened into more like a mile across, down past the cookshack, which was at the bottom of the sundance grounds. Coming from town, one made a left into the driveway past a small front yard, to the old wood-frame farmhouse. Just opposite the house, on the other side of the gravel drive, was a huge cottonwood tree; four men with hands linked could not have compassed it. A *woluta*, or tobacco ties and red-cloth flag, had been tied around it, for Elmer had said it had a spirit living inside. Just barely east of the tree was the old wooden garage, with the shallow interior and the tall, wide doors built that way for horse and wagons or a buggy.

Every hallway and room of the house was small, almost cramped. One came in through the back door onto a mud-room porch and then into the kitchen. Turning left, one found the entrance both to the living room and the hallway that led to the bath, a tiny bedroom, and the laundry area. I remember there was a garret upstairs, but the cellar was just a big, square hole underneath the house—dirt walls, dirt floor. There was another back door past the laundry, and coming straight in that, one came into the living room. This took up about half of the ground floor. There was one tiny bedroom just opposite the entrance from the kitchen, and inside, Elmer had his little pipe-carving shop. Chunks of catlinite, an old worktable with a vise bolted on it, saws, files, and other carving tools, deer hides, stems, and wood for pipe stems were everywhere. Catlinite dust formed a fine red patina on every surface.

Leaving through the back door, you stood on a tiny step overlooking the backyard. To the extreme left, up against the tree line, was a storage shed where Elmer kept his tipi covers tightly sealed in garbage cans. The sun-dance things, extension cords, and a sometime portable generator were there too. Progressing right, next was the toolshed, in front of which was a huge cable spool that stood on its end to make a worktable. Next was the changing shed, which may have started life years ago as a chicken coop. Against its side, facing the house, was stacked the wood for the sweat-lodge fires. Some fifteen feet or so past the shed was the men's sweat, with benches made of two-by-tens and sections of logs for supports. Each bench had an empty coffee can at either end for cigarette butts. Same for the women's sweat, which stood to the south of the fire pit, which was almost centered between the two. The south end of the yard was treeless, with a good view of the prairie. Continuing around this semicircle, but now on the same side as the back of the house, was the ceremony house with its little wooden ramp and two-by-four railing. Inside was mostly empty, save for a small woodstove, lots of pillows and ashtrays along the walls, and Elmer's ceremonial things up above the area at the west end, where he'd set up his altar. Feathers, a staff, various paintings and Indian art, and a strange *canunpa*, a pipe with two long stems opposite each other, were also there.

Outside again, there was a shady space of some twenty-five feet between the ceremony house and the farmhouse, and there were set up the two big picnic tables for socializing, *wopila* (thanksgiving feasts), or just sitting on in hot weather.

Just across the yard, between the toolshed and the changing shed, was a tall wooden beam about six feet long attached at either end to two uprights set in the earth. I was never sure if it had been a hitching post for visitors' teams, but Elmer used it to air his buffalo robes in the sun.

On one of my first times inside the ceremony house with Elmer, I had noticed the double-stemmed pipe and exclaimed to him, "I've never seen a *canunpa* like that before!"

He smiled, with an edge to it, and said, "That's how it works. You respect that pipe, could keep you from dyin' if you really sick. You don't respect it, could put you six feet under." I'd been learning the fire keeper's responsibilities, and in ceremony, I'd sort of made myself responsible for sageing the food—that is, ensuring that each item, and drinks, were adorned with a sprig of the white sage that grew so abundantly in the area.

But to finish the layout: The gravel drive became a dirt road as it reached the back side of the backyard. A short spur led up behind the house to the changing shed, for trucking in wood and rocks. The other portion led directly opposite this, past a final shed, which held the electric pump over the well that supplied the place with water. Then Patti's vegetable patch, (always in need of weeding), then down perhaps a quarter mile past a small cornfield on land leased to a local farmer, then through a thick woods of cottonwood and ash that gave out onto the sun-dance arbor. The dance grounds and cookshack were to the right of the road as one faced away from the house, while the parking and camping areas were on the left, or west side. Beyond the cookshack, the land fell away even lower to a really thick tangle of shrubs, tall cottonwoods, and more ash trees. There were one or

two *hanblechiya* sites down there, but mostly people going up on
the hill were driven across the road, past the meadow, up to much
higher ground among the hills, which were what the bluffs along
the road became.

But the grounds were like a beautiful park. Everywhere on
Elmer's place was tended meticulously. In the evening when the
rest of us were gathered around the TV, Elmer would go out into
the backyard. He had a little sickle blade welded onto the end of
a golf club shaft, and he'd go after any encroaching weeds, grass
that was too tall, and the like. I recall remarking once to Patti
about how he just always kept at it. "He said to me once," Patti
replied, "'My work's the only thing that keeps me going.'"

There was more to that statement than was obvious at first.
He also meant that as long as he followed the directions he'd been
given by the spirits about going up on the hill, they'd help him.
Elmer never talked about the spirits much. But he would often
relay messages from them. "The spirits, what they told me" was a
frequent prelude to many of his speeches. This is why he mostly
called himself an interpreter, the old term for medicine man. He
could speak the old-fashioned Lakota the spirits speak.

But to finish the description, the sun-dance arbor itself was
a double ring of ash crutches set with about a five-foot-wide lane
running between them, along the circumference. This was set
with openings at the points of the compass. The interior of the
circle was one hundred to one hundred twenty feet across. At
the west end was the gate that formed the entrance to the shade
arbor, a rectangular enclosure about fifteen by twenty. The north
and south gates were smaller, but the east gate was fairly wide
since it was through this that the sun-dance tree was brought
in. The trees had been cleared back from the ring, but I imagine
dancing at Santee was easier than dancing at Elmer's old place
in Ironwood at Rosebud, since that dance circle was set upon a
hilltop. At Santee, no matter where one was in the ring, there was

always a little shade, at least part of every day. During the four days of purification, the long stringers set on the crutches were covered with a roof of pine boughs, and the four walls of the rest area were almost completely enclosed. The drum and PA system were set up near the south gate, with the speakers on the arbor at various points. There was a further delineation of the inner circle made up of hundreds of short wooden pegs thrust in the ground that no dancer was to step across and no supporter or sing-er-drummer was to enter. After the tree went up on the fourth day, no water was allowed in the camp.

Speaking of water, the flood had contaminated every well on low-lying land in that part of the reservation, but we didn't know that yet. What we did know, Dave and I, as we went into the grounds on the second night after the flood, was that every earth-worm in that very rich soil had come to the surface and drowned as the waters rose. The stench was unbelievable. I almost lost my dinner a time or two and finally exclaimed, "Feh!"

"Yes!" Dave exclaimed. "This is *feh!*"

Earlier that day, Elmer, Dave, and I had been putting the cookshack back to rights, which meant loading the old burned-out fridge onto a pickup, hauling it out, and then going back into the brush and fishing out the three hundred-pound propane tanks. The current had washed them all some hundred yards north of where they'd been. Once we'd slid them back through the mud, I showed off a bit by picking up one that was almost full and walking with it a couple of steps, before my foot slipped out from under me in the slime and I had to let it fall. Elmer and Dave were watching me, and Elmer said, "Muscleman. I could do it too, once, but not anymore."

The big canvas tent Nico and I had gone to the Twin Cities for was almost a complete loss. We'd gotten it half erected a night or two before the flood on a pair of heavy posts. Now it was water-logged and caked with black, clinging mud. I tried once to get

underneath the part still above ground, but trying to lift it in
the stagnant, fetid, worm-polluted air was more than I could do.
I remember the night we'd tried to raise it, Patti was down there
with me and Nico, and I'd climbed up onto the crosspiece, some
ten or twelve feet up. Nico said, "Karl, you look like a big white
buzzard up there," and Patti had burst out laughing. There was
almost something malicious in her voice, but if you're going to be
around Indians, I knew, you've got to be able to take the teasing.

About this time, a week before sun dance, we got word from
the tribal council and the county that the floodwaters had over-
spread quite a large area, and all wells in low-lying areas had
been declared unfit for use. We hadn't noticed, because everyone
drank coffee, which was made in a big restaurant-style Bunn
coffeemaker. Dave commented, "That should be all right; those
things heat the water up to about three hundred degrees, which
is what it takes to sterilize it." It was OK to shower with, but the
Santee tribal council authorized the release of emergency funds,
and the tribe began hauling water, in every conceivable type of
container, out to folks all over that part of the rez.

By now, just before purification, a lot of people had come in
and set up camp. We set up the PA system for the meetings in the
evening. During these, Elmer, Patti, sun-dance leaders, and whoever wanted to speak would get up and get on the microphone.
I recall one young man who spoke before my first dance back in
1997. He had been diagnosed with lung cancer sometime previously—but it was now better, even, than being in remission. He
described his doctors as being dumbfounded, since they'd seen
that his damaged lungs were regenerating. "That's because I've
been praying with my *canunpa*."

There was also the story of the Native couple who had been
unable to conceive. They'd come to Elmer's sun dance, and I
think the husband danced while his wife prayed at the tree. They
were able to have a baby the next year.

Then there's the story of what had happened after my own first sun dance with my ex-wife—the healing of spina bifida and spontaneous draining of fluid on the brain of the little daughter of a Kiowa Vietnam vet, Jimmy, and his wife. The doctors at the VA hospital in Huntsville couldn't believe it. That healing had taken place so fast the little girl was out of the hospital and back home by the time we got back to Alabama.

In 1998, I believe, Elmer had gotten on the mike and told us all how he'd come to be an interpreter, or medicine man. It seems he was working as a feedlot hand on a big cattle outfit located on leased land on the Rosebud reservation, not far from the town of Parmelee. At that time, in the 1980s, he was still married to his first wife, Blanche, was drinking, and had eight kids, four sets of twins. One day, he told us, he heard a voice speaking Lakota, saying, "Come up to see us." He knew who it was, but he didn't go; he kept on working and drinking. A little while later, he heard it again and still wouldn't go up on the hill. One morning shortly after that, one of the sets of twins was sick, and they were dead by nightfall. At that point, even though he was drunk, his relatives intervened, put him through the sweat lodge, and put him up on the hill.

That was when the doctoring spirits came to him and said, "Good thing you came up; if you didn't, we were gonna take your whole family." They gave him his altar and the songs to go with it, and they told him to "put up a sun-dance grounds for the people." The principal spirits were Coyote and Iktomi, the tricky spider of Lakota mythology. He told us how one of the spirits had said to him, "I'm gonna be your buddy. Wherever you go, I'll be with you." And this was true. Time and again, I've heard that old man talk about events at sun dance, and elsewhere, that he could not have witnessed—like the time during the dance in 1999 when one of the dancers thought he could get away with smoking a cigarette in one of the outhouses. The next rest break, Elmer got up and told about it.

He also told us important things about the pipe, such as, "Some if they pick up the pipe and then later put it down, they don't go much farther." And, "Some, what they do, it isn't right. They might get mad and tell you, 'Oh, I'm pretty mad with you. I'm gonna take my *canunpa* and pray against you.' It doesn't work like that."

Well, I didn't do that, but when I think of the mistakes I've made since and how badly I behaved when I was being tested—as I see it now, I'm just amazed to still be here.

The memories have come back in a flood as I write this. I remember seeing Dave in the sun-dance arbor with his huge bald eagle feather. I remember Nico getting his eagle-bone whistle rammed up into his soft palate by the elbow of another dancer. I remember lying down in the arbor during one of the rest periods and starting to doze off and then having my nose tickled by an NDN guy with a long sprig of sage who'd sort of appointed himself the watcher. I remember overhearing a conversation between two other dancers about a really young medicine man who'd been running ceremony in some other rez town—and doing well for a while, but now, they said, he just wandered around town, laughing to himself. "Something must have happened." And I remember Elmer himself leading us in the dance at the end of the fourth day, when we all stank and were tired and so hungry! In his ankle-length dancer's skirt, carrying his golden eagle-wing fan, wearing his chief's headdress of bald eagle feathers, dancing to the drum, it almost looked like there was nobody inside all that regalia—as if it was a spirit who was leading us. Dancing three times toward the east gate, stopping a little farther on each time, and then the call of "*Hoka!*" going up as we finally charged out of the circle. As he once said to Dave and me, "If being an Indian was easy, everybody'd be doin' it!"

That sun dance of 1999 was the second year Elmer found himself unable to be out there dancing with us. Apparently years ago, when he was a competition dancer in the men's traditional category, he'd had a run-in with a sore loser. As he described it, this fellow, a Cherokee man, was angry that Elmer had beaten him out of the first-place prize. This was someone who still knew some of the old ways but wasn't too wise in using them. Elmer said this guy had put some bad medicine in his knee. He had taken something, like a little bone, and blown it into the joint. Ever since then, Elmer's right knee had given him trouble, and in his weakened state after the stroke and the attack by Shorty, he still tried, but he couldn't get past the first round. He was forced to supervise from the shade arbor, except for the piercings, for the rest of the four days.

I remember during purification, perhaps the first or second day, I was down by the dance grounds with Patti. Elmer and I had gotten the tractor stuck in the mud the day before, and we had the walkie-talkies to be used by security with us. Patti had called us once, and Elmer had said to me, "Don't tell her we're stuck!" We managed to get free with the help of a massive jack. But it was getting so you had to watch yourself around Patti. Her temper was getting worse. Anyway, we were watching the placement of a load of gravel at the lower intersection, between the cookshack, the camping and parking areas, and the sun-dance circle. It was still pretty gooey in spots that would shortly be heavily trafficked. I was describing to Patti the strange pain I'd felt in my chest the day before, or perhaps it was that morning. She said it was a sign from the grandfathers that I was going to pierce that year (i.e., in a few days). I had pretty much taken that as a given, without having thought about it too much. She said that she'd had several such experiences.

One other memory from purification comes to mind. There were by now a number of people showing up every day, local folks from Santee, besides Dave, Jamie, Nico, and myself. One afternoon, there were a bunch of us guys sitting out back around the big cable-spool table with Elmer. We'd just unloaded and stacked a big load of firewood, and I went up to the house and wandered back a little while later to find it'd turned into a stag meeting. The subject was pussy, and as I sat down, Elmer turned to me in a whirl and snapped, "You! You know what pussy is?!"

Everybody cracked up while I made some kind of affirmative response, being tempted to double down on his teasing by shaking my fist up and down with a stupid grin on my face, but I didn't.

"First year, when you get some pussy, make you so happy," Elmer said. "Next year, get kicked out." This last being a reference to my situation of being told to vamoose repeatedly by my own Cherokee spouse, which was how I ended up in Niobrara, Nebraska, with nothing else to do in the first place!

Well, the teasing went on for a while longer, and I've often wished I'd gone ahead with my own joke, but something Dave said to Nico later on has stayed with me. Dave was there when the joking was going on and was telling Nico about it.

"Grandpa was teasing Karl?" Nico asked.

"Oh! He wouldn't let go of Karl!"

"Well," Nico said. "He wouldn't tease you if he didn't like you."

During my first year, I remember pulling a watch of security duty at the main entrance. This was between the house and the sun-dance grounds, just at the margin of the woods. There was the cornfield between the road and the creek and a fringe of trees on the other side, between the dirt lane and the county road. We had driven hard to get there in time for purification from Alabama and were a bit beat. I recall that the husband of one of my ex's closest friends had come out to where I was on duty with a cup of coffee he described as "pretty stout." It was! So much so,

I couldn't finish it. But it kept me up for the business of smudging every vehicle that came in with a coffee can full of coals and cedar chips and tying a strip of colored cloth onto the aerial to show they'd passed in. There wasn't much to do with the walkie-talkie except run radio checks, which was good. No incidents that year. I remember 1997 as being the dance with the most attendees. People were camped all over the place, the weather was perfect, the atmosphere was joyous but restrained, and everything seemed so well organized. My only experience of weirdness came when I was going into the sweat lodge during the first day of purification. There were a lot of guys waiting to sweat and room in the back, so I said something like, "Why don't you guys scooch over a little?" No response. Mute, hostile stares. Then Larry Sellers—the *heyoka* who played the guide in the *Wayne's World* film—comes in, looks around, and just motions with his arm to tighten up, and you never saw such a hurry to comply! Message: "We'll take it from one of our own, white man, but not from you." Oh. OK, fine!

Back to 1999. After sun dance was over, there were traditionally supposed to be four days of rest for the dancers. Things weren't so tight economically then as they've become since. Quite a few folks stayed around for a day or two to help with cleanup, take down the sun-dance tree, dispose of it according to Elmer's directions (which is actually done after the end of the dance on the fourth day), and clean out the cookshack. A lot of folks deliberately left food behind for Elmer and Patti for the coming year. I recall, on about the fourth and last day of rest, a group of the last to leave brought up a whole pickup load of stuff from the cookshack and took an equal load of bagged garbage out with them. They left all the stuff on the concrete step at the back porch door. I remember feeling a little burned out, like maybe I'd been there and helped out long enough. Then Elmer came back up to the house from one of his tours of inspection. "Gonna look around," he'd say.

His eye fell on a nice-looking jar of preserves, and he and I began bringing the things into the kitchen. "Gonna eat that," he remarked, hefting the jar. I was suddenly overtaken with a realization of these peoples' lives. Here was this old medicine man, following his vision, maintaining sweat lodges for ceremony every month of the year, welcoming visitors onto his property, running ceremony—which entailed a lot of effort on the part of a seventy-eight-year-old man who'd just survived a major stroke—staying up 'til two or three in the morning while the spirits came in and doctored those who'd come for it, surviving an attack by an evil spirit, and then directing the complex and spiritually fraught ceremony of the sun dance! There he was, uncomplainingly gathering up the leftover flour, sugar, coffee, cooking oil, and miscellaneous items and planning on living on them—and to keep on doing this for as long as he could. Being an interpreter for the spirits is not something you can just retire from. I began to feel, having no real plans of my own, that I could probably stay on and continue to help out for a while longer.

So now, with sun dance over and the well hopelessly contaminated, the search was on to find a new homesite. The Santee Sioux was a checkerboard reservation. This means, out of all the land taken from that originally given to the Ponca, and then to the Isantee after the uprising in Minnesota, various "reforms" had been enacted over the years. Always pitched as incentives to "civilize" the Indians, and always resulting in a loss of their land base, these acts had resulted in part of the reservation being tribally owned, some tribal lands being leased to private stockowners through the BIA DLM arrangement, some being individual and family allotments, and some having been sold to non-Indians.

Elmer's main concern was that the new place have somewhere suitable for a sun dance. Patti, being an enrolled tribal member,

had a right to live anywhere she could on the rez. I remember
Patti being on the phone a lot with her family and quizzing me
about Jimmy Carter's Habitat for Humanity. In a couple of weeks,
with the tribe still trucking a couple of hundred gallons of water
per week, she'd found a promising spot—an old farmstead, part
of which had been bought back by the tribe recently. The white
family who had lived there had died out or left, abandoning
the place. On the north side of the main highway, as opposed to
where we were, on the south, this place was very remote, even by
rez standards, with no other buildings in view for miles.

PART 2
Santee, 1999

CHAPTER 4

The Spirits Like It Here

THE GRAVEL COUNTY ROAD, WHICH WAS THE ONLY WAY IN, took you to the bottom of the draw where the house and buildings were—with nothing in view but two rolls of the prairie. It was isolated. And it was like stepping back into the 1930s. The whole place was comprised of some fifty or sixty acres, and the farmhouse was set almost at the bottom of the narrow flat between the two hills of prairie ridge, which ran parallel for a mile or more, from east to west. The main driveway also ran between them for perhaps a half mile from the county road. As the land sloped downward from east to west, there was a stand of cottonwood, ash, and scrub as the land began to level out. This marked the beginning of the old farmyard. Behind the house to the west ran a little creek between steep, high banks. A small earthen bridge crossed the creek, just upstream (which was north) of the house. On the far side, the land rose sharply to the north and continued sloping downhill to the south. On the small patch of level land on the far side stood the huge old barn.

I remember being in there once with Elmer on an early tour and noticing that the feed stalls, or stanchions, were higher on one side, for the horses, and lower on the other, for the milk cattle. We learned from Patti that the family had lived there since before Prohibition, and it was so isolated because it had been the home of the local moonshiner!

The whole arrangement of the farm was multileveled. At the eastern end of the level patch, just as the lane emerged from the trees, there was a little wagon shed set up on the bottom of the northern ridge. South of this, the terminus of the southern ridge gave out on a narrow stretch of level land set somewhat below the level of the farmhouse. We ended up moving the ceremony house there.

Below the ceremony house site, south of and behind the house, was a more modern garage, maybe built in the late 1940s. Below this and the house, the land sloped down to the creek, but shelved a bit, and on this was a large shed. It had obviously been used as the main workshop of the farm, based on the many generations of fragmentary equipment lying half buried around it. Due west of this, past the farmhouse with its fenced-in yard, a little trail led up the slope of the north ridge to the old hog barn, another structure still standing, with most of the roof on. Just outside the farmyard, on the flat, was a large concrete slab due east of the house that had obviously been the foundation of some building. It was too small to have been the chicken coop. We guessed that was where the old man had probably kept his still. Down along the creek were huge old cottonwoods, and the whole place was choked with some forty years' worth of underbrush and overgrowth. The sandier soil of the farmyard supported so many varieties of burr—sand, cockle, and the tiny ones—you couldn't go in there without having your clothes completely clogged.

The first time we all trooped over there to have a look, Elmer said, "The spirits like it here."

I had taken a short family visit right after sun dance. I told them I'd be back on such-and-such a morning, but I was late. I kind of lollygagged on my way back, and didn't Patti light into me when I got back! "Where you been? Do you know Elmer's over there workin' alone? He wouldn't wait anymore! 'Where's Karl? Where's Karl?'"

I didn't have too much to say, just got over to the new place.

The house seemed ruinous at first, but with two large holes in the roof, the structure was actually in pretty good shape, considering. So we set about clearing brush and moving tools over in preparation to rebuild. The first thing was to clear brush from the farmhouse end of the drive, which was in good enough shape not to need grading. The next task was to get the number off the power pole so we could call the power company and get the electricity back on. This allowed me to move my homemade camper van over there and get my fridge, heater, and little TV going. Thus I became the de facto night watchman. Elmer and Pete (who'd returned after sun dance) would arrive about nine thirty in the morning, bringing two pickup loads of tools and stuff from the old place. I still went back over nearly every evening to have supper and shower, but most of my time was spent out there. It's one of the most isolated spots in the American outback. The nearest neighbors were at least five miles away, there was no phone service, and no cell phone service at that time or in that place. How very often I've wished I were back there. It was beautiful. The autumn prairie, the endless vista, the pears ripening on the ancient tree next to the drive, the utter stillness at dawn.

Since the chainsaw, power tools, and push mower were the first things we had to have over there, one of my first memories of the work there is of cleaning out a ditch and short culvert that entered the yard at right angles to the drive. I found my very first black widow spider.

Soon after our first tour, the Germans had come back from visiting Pine Ridge to see the new place. I took off from the old house with them in the back of the pickup I was driving. At that time, unfortunately, I'd only been over there once and couldn't find my way. We spent a little over an hour searching until I spotted a landmark (the peak of the barn) off through the trees and brought us in. Elmer and Patti had meant for me to wait for them to lead us, so they were there already. Patti was looking fire arrows at me, but Elmer just laughed. I apologized to my passengers and received a mild interrogation from Patti, but with others present, she didn't take it too far.

By now, it was late August, and the first order of work after clearing the road had to be clearing brush. We spent two weeks clearing the bottom of the drive, the farmyard, and the little fenced-in yard. The house was a two-story affair, built compactly, with a full-size cellar. The main door opened off the old kitchen, facing east into the yard, toward the bottom of the drive. The front door opened into the main room and was on the south side, facing a fringe of trees that grew at the lip of the ravine, which ran downhill behind the garage and in back of the big workshop. Once we'd cleared out the yard and mowed (an all-day task in itself), I remember we used a long rope and a pickup in four-wheel drive to pull off the old porch roof over the front door. It was a wreck, half collapsed already.

Along with numerous other items, cuttings, and trimmings, it went to become part of a huge burn pile in the gully behind the garage. The film *The Blair Witch Project* had just come out on the cable and satellite movie channels, and one of the first visitors remarked on the similarity to the house in the film, the location, and general creepiness. But we were changing that.

I remember pulling many empty cans of Butter-Nut Coffee, a now extinct brand out of Omaha, from the shop. The cans brought back to me an old TV jingle from childhood: "Three Cs on my report card / Oh boy, I'm in a rut! / I'll tell my Dad / But not until / He's had his Butter-Nut!"

But, to backtrack, that first afternoon after my trip, Elmer and I took a thorough inspection tour of the house, cellar, and garage. I recall going through the ground floor once with him, past the rotting floor in the kitchen hall, under the biggest roof hole, and remembering what he'd said about the spirits liking it, I put down one of my American Spirit cigarettes on the floor of a little back room, past the dining room. Just a general offering to what spirits might linger. On our return trip, Elmer spotted it, turned to me, and said, "You done that!"

"Yeah, I put it down for the spirits here," I told him.

He was pleasantly surprised, almost delighted, although that was all he said about it.

Then we went upstairs and found where a family of raccoons had been living for about the last twenty years. I recall seeing the tufts of fur everywhere, and you couldn't miss the huge pile of droppings just past the point where the roof was gone.

"Is that dirt? Or shit?" I asked him.

"That's shit!" he said, hesitating just a little at the obscenity.

We were just getting to the point in our friendship where we were getting over the formality (of politeness) and getting comfortable with a freer mode of expression. Elmer hardly ever used bad language, at least in English. His whole demeanor was too much the old-time Indian for that.

It was that same day, while we were still downstairs, that I discovered an old skeleton key hanging on a nail behind one of the doors. I gave it to Elmer, who popped it into his shirt pocket. It was the same room I'd left the cigarette in. After our tour upstairs, we went down into the basement.

The furnace was what I expected: a huge cast-iron "octopus" coal or wood burner. It was so big that the smoke pipe to the chimney was eight inches in diameter. The thing looked functional. Short of taking a sledgehammer to one, there's not much you can really do to it. The rest of the basement was as much a shambles as the rest of the house—piles of furniture broken for kindling and coal dust a half inch thick on the concrete floor. But under an old washtub in a corner, Elmer found an old, sealed, unlabeled whiskey bottle filled with a clear fluid. If there'd been any doubts about this having been an old moonshiner's place, the contents of that bottle laid them to rest! Talk about your white lightning! Neither Elmer nor I drank, of course, so he put the bottle, after we'd both sniffed at the contents, into a coffee can nailed to a wall. About halfway up the west wall of the basement, there was a two-inch-diameter pipe with a spigot on the end that, when opened, released a thin stream of water that quickly ceased. The location of the water supply for the place was one of our main concerns. Turned out, that was it, but we couldn't be sure it was reliable since the supply it offered was so meager. I remember mentioning offhand that I'd expected to find an old hand pump in the yard after we'd cut brush and mowed, but that never happened. There was a concrete slab out in the farmyard, just past the fence, with the family name and the year 1967 in it, but it was obviously a capped-off well, and we never broke it open.

By the middle of September, we were still cutting the last of the trees that overgrew the drive and farmyard. Elmer made sure to clear a lane behind the house so a vehicle could be driven completely around it if necessary. Then one day, he said he'd found something he'd been looking for! The second driveway.

CHAPTER 5

Bushwhackin'

THE MAIN LANE WE'D BEEN USING CAME OUT ABOUT TWEN-
ty-five feet north of the other driveway. The new lane
(which was probably older, according to Elmer) came over the
high ground all the way from the county road, then took a steep
plunge downhill at its terminus, which was in a direct line with
the back door of the house. It was completely overgrown, and no
one would have found it if they didn't know to look. The base
of the south ridge, before it swung away farther south from the
house, came in closest to the north ridge here, and it was over
this that the "new" lane ran. Looking east from the yard, you
could just make out its outline through the trees and brush—a
vehicle-wide depression that led between two low banks. Pete
and I had finished clearing out the lower road, and it fell to Elmer
and me to get after the new one. Of course, in such a remote
place, it only made sense to have an alternate way in or out.

There was an increasingly steep bank between the two roads,
and on the south-facing side of this, on the new road, there were
several small holes, well away from the house, about three or four

feet above the ground. "Them's coyote holes," he said. I couldn't believe it at first—the openings were only about six inches across! But he said, "Yeah, them's coyote."

This high road had to be cleared out completely, plus about eight feet on either side. It was to be the route along which a professional building mover would bring the ceremony house. We'd had ceremony on the new moon in September already, so this had to be done before the same time in October.

During the intervening time, Patti was on the phone a lot, taking calls from concerned parties, and we began to get an increasing stream of helpers and suppliers. Many of the names have escaped me, but as we began to get into the interior of the house—to take down the damaged walls and fix the hole in the hall floor near the kitchen—a fellow named Frank from Iowa City came and rewired the house, free of charge, and restrung the wire from the house to the power pole. Others came, including Jamie and Nico, to help strip off the old roof, and one older fellow came out with a free load of new roofing tin. I remember helping put on the new plywood roof, after the real carpenters had repaired the rafters, covering this with tarpaper, and then cutting and nailing on the new tin.

Before this, though, Elmer and I had finished bushwhacking the place and had moved indoors. I remember helping him strip off the interior walls upstairs. These were nothing more than flattened fifty-pound lard boxes nailed to the studs and wallpapered over. Under their lightly pasted coverings, the old blue logos were still bright. Indeed, I had confirmation of the age of the house; it must have been built in the 1920s, before the crash, when farmers were doing well. Not only were the two-by-fours really two inches by four inches, they were all of red oak—probably cut and milled locally. It's very hard to pull a nail out of one that had been there for eighty-odd years! Also, one of the old lard-box wall panels upstairs had a bright blue NRA sticker on it—and I mean the National Recovery Act of the early 1930s, with the light-blue federal eagle logo in use then. I should have saved that, but Elmer had told me to take all the trash material, especially the old plaster and lath from the walls downstairs, and use it to shore up the banks of the creek, especially around the earth bridge. There was a lot of erosion, and we had to prevent its loss.

But it seemed the more progress we made, and the more help we got, the more verbal and impatient Patti became. I recall she was really hot to get the new roof on. One morning, because of lack of crew, or short supply of roofing nails, I'd spent the time on other work. So about eleven, she pulls in, gets up in my face, and grills me as to what I'd been doing. When I told her, she snarled, "Everything but the roof, huh?!" This was just one example of her temper; unfortunately, there were to be many others.

About then, Elmer made another find. I've mentioned that there were various farm implements, and fragments of the same, scattered around the workshop below the house, but one morn-ing, Elmer and I went scouting up north along the creek trying to find a wellhead or some source of water. We didn't succeed, but tangled between two healthy saplings between the house and the hog barn, we came across an odd-looking piece of ironmon-gery—kind of like a big scoop welded out of a barrel-sized sheet of metal, with a framework and hitches rising above and in front of it. "We gotta get that!" Elmer said excitedly. "Cut it out!"

"Why?" I asked. "What is it?"

"That's an old snowplow from back in horse days."

"Oh, a real antique, huh?"

"Yeah, somebody could want it—pay money for it!"

So after lunch, I got out my little sixteen-inch chainsaw—or rather, oiled and gassed and sharpened it up some, as it was never really put away during the months I was there. Then I proceeded to cut the old scoop free, and of all the hard-to-get-to, lie-on-your-side-and-then-need-to-change-position-after-two-minutes-of-cutting kind of chain-saw jobs, it had to be number one! With the curved, half-barrel sides of the scoop rising on both sides and the trunks growing through part of the frame between them, it must have taken me nearly an hour to do ten minutes of actual cutting. But I got it free and dragged it down to the house yard. Elmer was pleased, but once again, the time had to be justified to Patti.

On another scouting trip to the north, earlier in the summer, we'd gone across the creek, past the old barn, and up onto the north ridge. This was close to the point where I'd mistakenly brought the Germans, and from there you could look out across miles and miles of northern Nebraska prairie, but turning, you couldn't see into the arrowhead-shaped yard below. The view was blocked by all the cottonwood, red elm, and ash trees along the creek. An ideal spot for a moonshiner, indeed. On that trip, I remember Elmer picked out a spot for the new sun-dance grounds, right up on a high saddle of land on that ridge. We went a bit farther downslope afterward, nearly a mile west of the house, and found a hillside containing rocks we could use in sweat. These didn't seem to be a local formation; rather they were deposits left when this area of the country had been scoured by the retreating glaciers. Possibly even millions of years older, when eastern Nebraska had been the shore of a vast inland sea, the Tethys. From where I stood, the endless crests and dips in the prairie looked exactly like waves, frozen in earth and time.

But I've gotten ahead of myself once again. Before all this, during the early days of the move, for a week or two, Elmer would show up first. We'd unload his pickup and get started doing something until Pete showed up. One day, Pete didn't come 'til late, and Elmer and I were out there on our own. As we finished with clearing out the last of the scrub growth in the farmyard, Elmer stopped and motioned me over.

"You see that?" he asked me, pointing to a strange lump resting in the fork of a small tree. "That's that *wanagi pejuta*, that ghost medicine you guys had to burn one time." He was referring to the attack by Shorty. "You get some o' that, burn it in your house, an' no ghost ever gonna come and bother you." I marked the fungus for later attention.

Also, early on in our rebuilding, a small lean-to at the very back of the house had to be taken off. As I pulled up the last of the boards that had supported it against the house, I counted six female black widow spiders, just lined up and sitting there. I disposed of the near rotten lumber with unusual care and then went to report my find to Patti. "Patti, there were six black widows under the last board I pulled out!"

"You didn't kill any of 'em, did you?"

"Oh no!" I said, shocked. "I hope I'd know better than that!"

A little later, when we were doing piecework on the roof, which was delayed several times while I drove twenty miles out and back to buy more roofing nails, Patti became just impossible. I remember how hard a time I was having one morning, pulling those rusty old nails out of that eighty-year-old red oak. We'd all been working on the new place every day for a month or more, with no breaks. Suddenly, the cheap hammer I'd just bought from a discount bin at a local hardware store bent double in my hands! And the head came off! I snapped! I remember I roared and cussed and flailed at the two-by-four I'd been bothering, then flung it down and went for my pickup without a word to anyone, except those choice few I'd left hanging in the air. I went up to Vermillion by myself for the weekend, as it turned out. Checked into a hotel, showered, and spent the time lounging on the bed watching movies and cartoons. Yes, Vermillion. I'm sorry, but it's true—I really was that hard up for entertainment. I ate at the Perkins next to the Super 8 and didn't call anyone.

When I went back the next Monday, Elmer just looked at me and started laughing. Pete asked me what the deal had been, but he was grinning too. I explained about the new hammer being just the last straw, and he told me all that stuff in those discount bins was junk. Patti came by earlier than usual and gave me a look but didn't say anything. Later, Pete took me aside again and said how what I'd done had turned out well. "Patti pulled us off the house that evening and took us into Santee for dinner at the casino!"

The dry weather continued that summer after the flood, and by the beginning of autumn, the nights were beginning to become quite cool. One cloudy weekend, we moved my little camper onto a patch I'd cleared in the woods behind my camper van. My van was just to the south, or in the trees to the left of the lower drive. I never did get moved into that unit, as it turned out, but I did make one discovery. While clearing out the space for the camper, my eyes caught a strangely regular shape, up on top of the south bank, just below the lip of the overland, or upper, driveway. When I was done, I went down to the house, where Elmer and some others were, and told him I thought I'd found the water. We went up there. There was a path through the brush, quite a narrow trail on the hillside in places, and came upon a circular stone-and-concrete structure some four feet high. It was at least six feet around and in a direct line to the house. When I crawled on top and lifted the wooden lid, there was water far below me. Hard to tell how deep, or how far down, but well below the level we stood at. We returned to the house, satisfied the mystery of the water had been solved, but it was not to be.

There was one old flush toilet in the house, and one of Elmer's followers was to come and replace the plumbing. I remember Elmer telling me to save the thick wax ring around the base. It looked so bad that I was gonna pitch it. We were taking up the stool, since most of the kitchen hall and bath had to be refloored. Before all this, though, we had to use one of the outhouses we'd carted over and dug a pit for. I remember on one trip with

Elmer and Patti, from the old place into town, I joked that when I'd crossed the Missouri on my trip to Vermillion, I'd seen the five-hundred-dollar outhouse that had been swept away in the flood, floating along. It was getting so that any time spent with Patti was just no fun, and I was trying desperately to put a little fun into things. She'd eased up a little, after my weekend retreat, but it didn't last.

Soon enough it was early October, and a couple of Elmer's sons (not Gilli) showed up to help out—Norman and his brother Webster, the youngest of the old man's kids. Norman helped out with this and that but didn't stay long. Webster was around for a few weeks. Just before then, however, one morning Patti decided to act out on her resentment of my independent action. Complaining about how long it was taking us to dismantle the wall along the kitchen hall, she picked up a hammer from behind me and, without warning, swung it into the plaster a few feet from my head! I shoulda decked her for it, but I didn't. Can't remember what she said exactly, I was so startled, then busy suppressing rage, but it was something along the lines of "Now we'll see something get done."

She pulled off a few square feet of old wallboard, and without bothering to scoop up what she'd done, she exclaimed at how hard the work was. Then she dropped the hammer and beat a hasty retreat.

My reaction, which I kept to myself, was, "Not as easy as it looks, is it, Patti?"

Now, before I move past the summer of that year, one or two other instances have come to mind, after writing of the time they occurred.

The first is from just before sun dance. Patti's son, Jamie, was having trouble with his girlfriend. They were living together, but on this day, that was at an end. He asked Nico and I to help him get his stuff and move. So we drove into Santee itself, past the rows of ugly little BIA/HUD prefabs, until we got to the right one. Then we loaded his things from the front porch, where she'd piled them. Jamie had lived for a while in the tiny upstairs garret in the old farmhouse, and his little daughter was around a lot. I heard Patti accuse him of having spoiled his woman by being too nice to her, but he didn't seem too upset by it all. He was a good singer and, as I've mentioned, frequently came to monthly ceremony to help.

Another time, during the move and rebuilding, Jamie had thrown my new Makita cordless drill onto a picnic table fairly roughly, and I kinda yelled at him not to. "It's just a Makita," he said, and then made me laugh by mocking my angry voice: "Rahr-rahr-rahr!" I'd been a little out of line; he hadn't hurt it a bit, and I've since come to appreciate his disparagement.

But Elmer was worried about him. Another day soon thereafter, we'd all convened in the inner farmhouse yard for lunch, and Elmer said, "What's Jamie gon' do later on after we're down here? Where he gon' live with that *wincincala* he got? Been thinkin' about that."

Yet again, on the afternoon when he and I had finished clearing out the high drive, after he'd pointed out the coyote holes to me, he suddenly reached down and picked up a small rock. It was unremarkable—small, irregularly shaped, black-and-white banded—but he seemed to be very pleased with it. "Heyoka stone," he said, showing it to me. Heyoka the contrary, the black-and-white thunder clown, the power in the west, which, if it comes to a man during *hanblechiya*, makes him contrary and a healer. He left and took the stone down to where we'd recently put up the first sweat lodge.

I recall during my first few years of sun dancing that there was a lot of misunderstanding from various Indians about Elmer. One fellow in Huntsville dismissed him as an old drunk who was selling ceremony. Another, who heard that Elmer was healing and doing ceremony with an Iktomi altar, declared that he was doing bad medicine. And it's true, when someone says of another, "He's Iktomi." It ain't never a compliment. But being a trickster isn't his only function. There are stories where Iktomi saves the people and others where he helps them. One of Elmer's songs goes, "All over the world / I come to help / A spider says this as he comes." And, Elmer would joke about it: "Sometimes I like to talk *heyoka*," meaning the opposite of what's said.

I finished clearing the loose brush out of the road and then hunted around until I found what I thought was the same kind of stone. I took it down to him, where he was setting up the old shop as a changing room and storage for his sweat things, but he didn't accept it. Just looked at me without saying a word. That was how I knew I'd messed up, when he got quiet like that.

It's impossible to keep events in their chronological order, but it was about this time (mid-October) that a bunch of sun dancers showed up with the roofing materials, electrical supplies, and new carpeting. The place really began to take shape. I recall taking down the old wainscoting in the living room carefully, since it was nice paneling. I numbered each piece in order and stacked it up outside. I also recall scouring the antique marts for a floor grating for the same room. The main vent was large, relying on convection from the furnace below, but it meant we had a big square hole to walk around in the middle of the main room. It was a pain having to work around a pitfall. It seems like, when it came time in the unfolding of what needed to be done, I got the fiddly jobs. This is part of what gave me such satisfaction in the work—it exercised my creativity. Finding a "new" grate that almost fit and then nailing in a good piece of wood to make it fit was easy. It was the step at the back door that was challenging.

The old step had probably seen the most wear of any part of the house over its lifetime. Now it was beginning to sag, and it crumbled a little every time you stepped on it. A definite ankle-busting hazard. So one afternoon when I found a length of old timber that looked right—finished on two sides with rounded edges along the long sides—I picked it. All that was needed was to cut it to length. Out with the chainsaw, and off with a slice from one end. Then I set it in place and stood behind it on the kitchen floor to pound it in with a sledge. Too tight, won't fit all the way. So I pried it out, sliced off just a hair, and recommenced pounding. Pete wandered by at this point and said, "Boy! That's sure some precision work!" He was kinda joking, but I kept it up and drove that step into place so tightly, there was no need to spike or nail it down.

Norman and Webster stayed around for a bit, but apart from Webster using a jigsaw to s-l-o-w-l-y cut out a new archway for the kitchen hall and laying a few floorboards, they didn't seem too committed. Just before this, a fellow named Thunder also showed up and brought his pressure washer with him. He was one of those "sun-dance followers," meaning he went around and helped out at different sun dances without being a dancer himself. He was a tall, blond, bearded, long-haired guy from Virginia or West Virginia. One of my most vivid memories is of him teasing Webster one morning, when Web had childishly sat himself down in one of our few chairs, after working an hour or two, and refused to do anything more. "¡Hola, *el jefe!*" said Thunder, calling him "boss" in Spanish. He stayed on 'til after we got the ceremony house moved over, and then he had to leave. Never got to pressure wash and repaint the house's exterior.

Patti was being more and more difficult. I think she may have driven Elmer's boys away. I'll never forget the time I had gone into Santee for lunch, takeout at the casino cafeteria, since we couldn't depend on her to keep us fed. Here she came just as I got back, with a big pot of stew and a plateful of fry bread. She gave me a dirty look and a little lip for getting lunch, never mind there was no way for us to communicate, even if we'd had cell phones.

Then she took the takeout containers of food—fries, burgers, and chicken strips for Elmer—and packed them home so she wouldn't have to cook dinner! Kinda outrageous, but you couldn't say anything to her.

Now that I'm recalling another incident at the new place, late in the summer, I think I must have been mistaken about us having moved an outhouse over there, at least at first. One afternoon, Elmer and I were over at the new place by ourselves; Pete had returned from his spree but was back packing up a fresh load of gear to bring over to the new place. Suddenly, Elmer grabbed a shovel and muttered something about having to go to the bathroom real bad. He went off into a clump of trees between the house and where the ceremony house was to be. When he came back, that's when he spotted the *wanagi pejuta* up in a tree.

Getting back to events that fall, though, one thing I've failed to mention is that during the years the farm had been abandoned, someone had turned it into a pot plantation. There were little patches of plants, and single ones everywhere, but not past the farmhouse. Around the house and farmyard, and especially across the creek in the old pasture in front of the barn, was the main field—huge stands of eight-foot-high female plants, and not left over from any WWII rope-making effort on the home front, either! On a hot September afternoon, I could smell the resin fuming off them. Also, someone had spray-painted "Alonzo's Party House" up in the hayloft. Probably the nephew of some tribal council member who was responsible for leasing the land out to whoever had run cattle on it for minimal BLM grazing fees and a healthy kickback. Patti had gotten a little of the property's history, but now it was once again tribal land.

Sometime in late October, Elmer and I went on a willow-cutting expedition. The house was coming along, despite Patti's complaints. The outbuildings and yard were all passable, and ceremony time was approaching.

We left together in Elmer's ancient Ford pickup, having loaded a hatchet and small brush saw for me, and Elmer's trusty Estwing small axe was already on board. Going out to the graveled county road, we went north toward Santee and stopped after about a half mile. It was a hike down to the bottom of the field, but Elmer found a way through all the furrows to a small but dense stand of osiers, or young willows. Except for the osiers, other scrub growth along the bottom, and the grass along the road, there was no standing vegetation. The fields were marked with postharvest stubble. A blue October morning sky gave over to a more Novemberish gray. It was the first really crisp day of the season, with the first frost perhaps a week or two away. He showed me two right sizes, longer and shorter, and we set to work.

It was a pretty thick stand; when we were on opposite sides, we couldn't see each other. We trimmed off the branches on the spot, and after we'd gotten some twenty-odd lengths, we loaded them onto his truck and went back.

Then the work began! Getting a long, heavy iron rod from the toolshed, Elmer and I first raked an area smooth and then dug a central pit, about two feet in diameter, and a foot deep in a circular space about fifteen feet across. Piling up the earth carefully to the west of the outer edge of the circle, he then took a wooden stake and twine and inscribed a circle about twelve feet across. Next he took the iron rod and made two deep holes, one inch in diameter and about four feet apart, along the west, north, east, and south. Then he told me to do exactly the same, only in between the first sets. While I was thus engaged, he began driving the longer of the willows into the first set of holes, at the cardinal points, always starting at the west. By the time I finished, he was too, or nearly, and we started work on the horizontal supports of the sweat-lodge frame.

There were three lower and heavier tiers, which included a piece hooped around the western uprights and tied to the lowest tier; this formed the doorway. The fourth tier, or crown, was a slender whip of an end, which Elmer bound into a circle with bark we'd stripped from other lengths. The sixteen uprights we bent and bound across, each one to its opposite so that the center was no higher than five feet or so. After the uprights and horizontals were bound together, using coat-hanger wire and pliers, Elmer lashed the crown with thin strips of bark. I'm not sure, but perhaps it was the addition of the crown that made it a real medicine lodge to be used for ceremonial purification.

All of this except the door, of course, was covered by a layer of heavy canvas, tied down with ropes. These went around the base, from one side of the doorway to the other, and ropes tied to this were strung across the top and knotted down tightly. The flap for covering the door was also tied across the top rope.

The last thing was that Elmer took the little pile of earth I'd dug up to form the pit and ran a little low ridge of it out a little ways from the front of the door, where it ended in a packed-down pile a couple of feet farther out. This of course was the spirit trail, and the hill was where the buffalo skull was to be set for the pipe rest. Elmer had the eagle-feather staff, a tall one, with its felt *woluta* and abalone shell already in place.

By the time the building movers showed up at the old place, most of Elmer's tools, gear, and sun-dance paraphernalia were either set up, in use, or stored at the new place. I remember one creepy episode, just before dark, the evening before I was to clear the road. A strange pickup showed up suddenly, coming in on the low road, no headlights, and did a quick one-eighty and skedaddled back up the high road. It was just some local white boys letting their curiosity get the better of them, but I got very defensive and territorial. I recall saying something about loading up the double-barreled twelve-gauge shotgun I'd bought from Elmer earlier in the summer. Pete kinda talked me down, telling me if I was serious, I should take out the loads in the shells, reduce the powder content, and reload with rock salt. That made me stop and think. I got a good look at the vehicle, and when I spotted it in Niobrara again, I gave the driver a very hard look and got a shit-eating grin in return, and that was the last we saw of them.

We went over the route the movers were to take, and on the morning of the move, I went out with my chainsaw to take down any and all overhanging limbs. It was the back way in, a turn off the highway farther east on a very empty stretch of road.

The house movers were a family-seeming team of some three men and a mom, who drove. It was really something watching the guys use huge hydraulic jacks to lift the ceremony house, set the long supports underneath, then jack it all up even higher until the big flatbed could back up underneath.

I took off in one of the pickups with my chainsaw and was at the new place, with all obstructing limbs down, well before they got there around noon. Elmer was driving his old blue Ford as a pilot car and was obviously pleased when he arrived. He got out and told me, "Sit down, take a smoke. Now you gon' see somethin' you didn't see before."

We had a whole slew of concrete blocks ready, most of them taken from the old foundations, and it was impressive how the crew again backed the rig in, set up the support, jacked up the whole structure, drove the rig out, and set it down on the positioned blocks just as neat as you please.

It was about this time that the allergies and sinusitis I'd contracted earlier in the summer began to be a problem. I recall some weeks before sun dance, at the old place, I woke from a nap one afternoon with a weird sensation in my right ear—as if there were a cone of heat projecting out from it. I didn't know it then, but I was developing a sinus infection, which I ignored for the next few months, until it began to affect my blood pressure.

The stressful situation with Patti may have had something to do with that, as well. I remember that the morning after the first monthly ceremony at the new house, Nico's vehicle had broken down. Somehow, getting it back entailed me walking a long distance back to the house, from where I'd had to accompany him. This was back a mile or more, along the same route I'd just bushwhacked two days earlier. I recall being just dog tired, because ceremony had gone late. A few people were there, Nico, Jamie, Patti, her sister, and other relatives. Elmer had asked the spirits why he was getting weak, and they'd said, "You got nothing on your stomach." At which point, Patti had positively snarled at him, declaring she wasn't gonna do any extra cooking for him, or something angry, and like that.

Nico had spent a stretch in the Cherry County jail after sun dance. While we were looking to move and then moving, his ex-wife's parents in California had accused him of kidnapping his boy, whom he'd had at sun dance. I knew he'd been praying to get his family back together. I went and visited him there and at his request brought him string, tobacco, and some colored cloth to make prayer ties. The jail was strange. The upper walls of the main hallway were decorated, if that's the right word, with dozens of homemade pipes, bongs, and other dope-smoking paraphernalia the cops had seized over the years.

After we'd gotten the ceremony house set up and had ceremony, Thunder and I sat up one evening making the prayer ties prescribed by the spirits. He told me a few things about himself that had come up for him in ceremony. Elmer had talked about how some Lakota considered Jesus to be the first sun dancer, since he'd been pierced to a tree, at the base of which were seven stones—just as were used in the entrance sweats to sun dance. Thunder said, "Man, it took everything I had to keep quiet. I wanted to tell him, 'It wasn't like that.'" He believed he'd been present, as someone, at the crucifixion. Other than that, he was a perfectly normal-seeming guy. On Sunday morning, we had strong black coffee in the ceremony house, where he'd slept after ceremony, and he said he'd soon have to be on his way.

And I had problems of my own. I had been a pot smoker for many years, although I'd cleaned up on my own, months before coming to Santee the first time in 1997. The first frost was only a week or so away, if that, and all those plants in the pasture were talking to me. I wasn't the only one Patti's abuse was getting to; she told me that on my last away trip, Pete had gotten into the garage and drank the bottle of moonshine we'd found in the basement. Elmer had come to her and said, "Pete's drunk."

Nonetheless, he was in high spirits for the first sweat before ceremony at the new place. Before the men went in, Elmer and some of the older men were talking about how during our life on this earth, "We don't know it, anything. By the time we get to know something, we gonna kick the bucket."

As I've said, Elmer asked the spirits why he was feeling so weak, and they said that it was because he had nothing in his stomach, which made Patti freak out because she took it as a reproach for slacking on her duties and not feeding everyone well. Patti had been shown up by the spirits and hadn't liked it. From that point on, it was walk-on-eggshells time whenever she was around. For her to have yelled at a medicine man, her man, in ceremony like that was the depth of bad manners. She was getting the same attitude toward the men as toward the dogs, all of whom were starting to look a little thin. On the way into that first ceremony, I remember Florian Bluethunder was walking over with a bread bag full of sandwiches for the feast afterward, and Waziya came up in the dark and ripped it out of his hand.

I remember one lunchtime when Patti had come in and Elmer, Pete, and I were sitting in the living room about to eat. We could see Patti was winding herself up to go off on another tirade. Pete got up and said something about there being fewer flies outside, and that got him out of it. I wished I could go with him, and the next moment, the breeze had blown a sheet of newspaper she had up and over her head. I started giggling, but all she said was,

"Karl sure liked that," in a threatening tone. And then she went off on us—can't even remember what about.

About a month later, after the interior was mostly rebuilt—new carpet in, rewiring done, roof on, tools almost all over from the old place—Elmer and I had been working all morning and had just gotten back from another hunt for the source of water when Patti pulled in. She just lit into the old man, didn't even get out of the car. Elmer was trying to explain what we'd just done, but it was no good. Later, I happened to pass by the kitchen door, looked downstairs, and he was just sitting by himself in the basement, looking like a whipped pup. From then on, I hated Patti.

I kept to my own way that time, although I felt an urge to get myself down there with him and at least commiserate. But I talked myself out of it, feeling embarrassed for us both and convincing myself that there was really no practical solution to the situation. Patti was the enrolled tribal member, and the house and land were in her name, so there was little we could really do but grin and bear it. I'd been sort of planning on staying on indefinitely, but I was beginning to long for escape.

Speaking of embarrassment, I must now come to the confessional part of this remembrance. Early one morning in mid-October, before anyone else had shown up, I was out scoping the marijuana crop. I was across the creek, away from the barn, at the edge of the pasture by the creek, staring at that particularly fragrant and tall female plant. The first frost was imminent, and I knew that once the frost touched it, all those pounds and pounds of pot would be lost. The thought of the waste was what really got me. Without touching that plant, I went out and bagged a dozen or so medium-sized plants' worth, stuffed 'em in two paper sacks—but I didn't smoke any. I like to think I abstained out of respect for the old man. However, later that day, I was up on the north hillside, cutting brush below the hog barn, and suddenly I felt this presence. I looked up, and there was Elmer, staring straight at me, standing in the exact spot I'd been that morning. Our eyes met, all the way across the creek, and I looked away first. That was the thing about being around a *wicasa wakan*: There were simply no secrets. Anything that happened that might affect him or his, the spirits would know about it and would tell him. He'd know who was off smoking a cigarette in the outhouse during sun dance, and there was no other explanation for it. He'd made that accusation on the PA, without naming names, and no one lied to him. It would have been ludicrous: "No, I wasn't!"

I've kept this to myself 'til now, but at the beginning of that first monthly ceremony, when I was done with my usual chore of making sure a sprig of sage was set in place with each dish and drink, as a blessing, he grinned at me and said, "You got something on you mind." It was true; those little sacks of pot were beginning to weigh on my conscience, but not as much as having been found out.

So there they stayed, untouched in my van for the next two or three months. Since I've rehearsed this justification in my mind so many times since, I may as well get it out on paper. If you were to take an alcoholic who'd been on the wagon for three years or so, and who'd cut out his associations with his former drinking buddies and been kicked out by his soon-to-be ex-wife, and then get him in a position where the verbal abuse is beginning to become eerily reminiscent of his failed marriage—and further, the only job he can get is night watchman at the local brewery—well, you tell me what's going to happen! For years afterward, though I didn't fall back into regular using until sometime in 2002 or 2003, that was my excuse and rationale.

But by the week after the first monthly ceremony at the new place, the house was livable, except for the transport and connecting of the kitchen stove. At one point earlier in the summer, I'd allowed Nico to shanghai me away so we could go and pick up a vehicle of his. I ended up spending nearly two days away, and when I got back to the old place, I apologized to Elmer for being gone a day. "More like two," he said. So when Patti gave me a job I really wasn't up to, I figured Nico owed me a favor.

It was about this time that the health problems I'd had earlier in the summer began to be an issue. I didn't know it, but my sinusitis was being exacerbated by seasonal allergies and by my smoking. I didn't find this out until later, but my blood pressure was also spiking pretty high. So when Patti pretty much ordered me to sweep up all the old coal dust out of the basement, I had to ask Nico to fill in for me. It was a gray October afternoon, or early in November, and Elmer had left with Patti after she'd given me my marching orders. I recall somewhat desperately explaining my situation to Nico, who luckily was on-site that day, and he agreed. I was beginning to have funny turns, feeling weak, and almost dizzy spells.

I wish I could remember more of what Nico said to me then. He was a trickster, a charmer, and downright hilarious when he was at it. He did a great Master Yoda. Anyway, he helped me out that time, and I'm still grateful for it; breathing all that old mold and coal dust would've about killed me. But he would let me and the old man down later on. Nonetheless, he was a fun guy to be around and a good worker—and he covered his own expenses while he stayed with us at Santee.

A week or so later, just after the first frost, as the weather was beginning to have a real snap to it, I went into Niobrara for a visit to an optometrist's. I was about out of contact lenses. I was told my blood pressure was two hundred over one hundred twenty and that I needed bifocals. The doc said he could see the capillaries in my retinas were dilated when he went in to look and told me to get it seen to immediately.

By now, it was almost the new moon of November, which meant it was nearly time for monthly ceremony again. The days were still warm enough to work outside, and bright and clear. I'd mentioned something about a stressful work situation to the doc, and he'd offered to write me a note excusing me. But I turned him down, guessing (correctly) that it would make not a bit of difference to Patti. She hadn't been around too much since she'd gone off on Elmer for nothin', but one time she showed up just after lunch as I was sharpening everyone's knives for them. I've always appreciated a good knife and was carrying around a classic Buck in a belt sheath that summer. It wasn't too hard to learn to hone one to a good edge, and when Pete saw me take it out and begin with my oil and stone, he asked me to do his. Then Thunder asked, and so the three of us were sitting down when here comes Patti in the old Aerostar. The first thing she said when she got out was something accusatory about the crew wasting time, and she was dismissive when we tried to explain that, in the long run, sharp tools would make the work go faster. She just snorted. For a woman who was getting a house and grounds completely cleared and rebuilt for nothing—just in recognition of who her old man was—she was hard to please.

It was actually about now that the dogs were brought over, which means the knife-sharpening incident took place some few weeks earlier. Waziya and the yellow female came over in Elmer's or Pete's pickup, no problem, but no amount of coaxing would get Tegi into a vehicle. I finally had to pick him up, despite his tough-guy growling act, and he lost it. He was so scared of riding in a vehicle that everything that was inside him came up. Inside the first five miles, I swear half the contents of that animal's digestive tract came up, and I had to put up with the mess and stench the rest of the way and hose off the floor mats when we got there.

I recall it was during the preliminaries to the November ceremony while Elmer was setting up the altar that I began to doze off a little, and Jamie suddenly hit his hand drum a cracking good wallop, which jerked me awake. Nico said, "That just about made Karl jump out of his skin," which caused some friendly laughter. As usual, all the men were against the north wall, the women and kids on the south. As soon as the altar was up and Elmer started talking to us, even before the lights were doused, the kids were asleep. Every month, it was the same. The spirits would put the children to sleep the first thing they did. Sometimes, even before we started singing to call them in.

This was when, during his preliminary remarks and questions to us, Elmer said, "We use it, seven rocks in sweat for the sun dance. That's how they did it back in centuries, put seven rocks at the base of that cross."

That got Thunder's reincarnation panties in a bunch. I'd heard this kind of thing before, that some of the Lakota who'd been exposed to the Christian dogma regard Jesus as the first sun dancer. Although the two traditions are completely alien, the central idea—offering one's own suffering and blood to ensure the answering of prayers and continuation of life—is the same. I remember that one as a good ceremony. The spirits came in strong, and we didn't stay up too late, no more than 2:00 a.m. Also, after the ceremony was done and the feast was over, as the altar was being disassembled and put back in that suitcase, I relaxed a little too much and cut a small, loud fart. Again more laughter, and Patti said, "You relaxed a little too much."

Lorna, one of the lady sun-dance leaders, asked, "But how did you make it sound like it came from over here?"

"Ventriloquism," I replied. It fell flat. Not the boff I'd hoped for.

As to Thunder's semi-messiah complex, he told me that when he was five or younger, his mother, who was crazy, tried to drown him in the bathtub. Fortunately, his aunts had caught her and rescued him. They promptly took her out to the yard and, according to Thunder, beat the shit out of her and told her if they ever caught her doing it again, they'd kill her. I detected a little overcompensation going on: Those who'd undergone such an assault on their self-esteem at such a young age might form a negative opinion of themselves, unconsciously, and would have to find something of themselves of supreme value to balance this. Such, anyway, was my undergrad psychology take on it.

It was now the third week in November, the Saturday that hunting season began. It was a little unnerving at first, hearing rifle shots in the middle of the afternoon and not being able to see the source or even tell where they were coming from. Any loud sound bounced around between those two ridges in a way that seemed like it could be coming from anywhere. It was impossible to gauge distance too. I remember one morning, a couple of Santee guys came down the low road and stopped when they saw my camper. I was already up and had to tell them that the premises were inhabited now and they couldn't hunt there. One of them said that they'd been hunting there for years and that Patti was his auntie. When I mentioned this to Pete later on, he laughed and said, "Cuts no shit now. It's rez land again!" We started discussing a piece I'd heard on NPR that morning: Some idiot newly elected Republican had introduced a bill to terminate all the government's treaty obligations to all Native nations. "Hey," I said, "screw two hundred–plus years of American legal history! I'm a neoconservative. I don't care. I don't have to honor the treaties!"

"Fine," said Pete. "You don't want to keep up your end of the agreement, just give the land back."

Sometime during the next week, the phone company came in and ran a landline from the trunk out on the county road up to the house. After all the expenses of the move, money was apparently getting tight. Patti gave me the November power bill for the old place and the new installation and first month's charges, even though I was already contributing quite a lot, if I may say so. I remember she was pretty "here, you pay this" about it, and I felt burned. I'd made multiple trips to the building supply store in Niobrara and elsewhere when they ran out of the special roofing nails—and I was doing literally nothing else but helping out, plus feeding the crew lunch most days. What with one thing and another, I was getting that ready-to-go feeling again.

Something Elmer said in ceremony that month has stayed with me: "Karl's done quite a bit of work, but I always gotta keep my eye on him." I seem always to strike others as an eccentric, the absent-minded-professor type—a space case, not to put too fine a point on it. Though that stung a little, Patti unexpectedly came to my defense. She was kind of getting after some of the local folks who'd come, her Isanti relatives, for not helping out more. After joshing with them about how she was "cracking the whip" over us guys, she spoke to them rather sharply about how no one ever brought in a load of firewood or rocks for the sweat lodge. Then she brought up the issue of the stolen generator. "Karl was watchin' the house while we were gone, and he went out and bought us a new one. And he's a white man." I just kept still and looked at the floor in front of my crossed legs. I was kind of embarrassed to be made the center of attention, but it was to happen once more.

At the end of that ceremony, as he always did, Elmer gave us our instructions for making our monthly ceremony ties. So many squares of cloth, in their several colors, in sequence, to be folded up with a pinch of tobacco inside, and all tied onto one long string. People who were doctored were given an additional set, plus they would have to put up *wopila*, or make thanksgiving ties and flags, donate a feast, and do a giveaway. As he always told us, "If we make them ties, the spirits, they gonna help us. If we don't, they won't." And, "That's what we need, on this Mother Earth, good health and help." *Wicozani* and *wowoke*. Somehow, I hadn't yet gotten into the habit of making them. But the next evening, Thunder was hanging out in my camper with me, watching TV, and he got me started by saying, "Well, after we make our ties, things'll smooth out around here." I'd kind of been bending his ear about Patti. That chance comment got me started doing it, made me realize I needed to, and I've been making them every month ever since.

I hadn't been in for a doctoring for myself in ceremony for the sinusitis and hypertension, but it seemed like just being there, and especially drinking that doctoring drink Elmer brewed up every month, helped. I was beginning to suffer from the stress of having to be around Patti. Things would go along smoothly for a week or so, and then she'd erupt over anything. After the phone was in and the new carpeting down, it was my job to replace all the old oak wainscoting around the base of the living room. I remember going into Niobrara for a tack hammer and a box of long tacks. Thankfully, I had numbered each piece of the stuff as we'd taken it up, so putting it back right was a snap. Another crew of Elmer's sun dancers had come in and drywalled all the walls about the time the ceremony house was moved, so that was done.

There was still a lot of brush to be cleared around the place, so one morning I went into town early to fill up my pickup and all the gas cans for the chainsaws. I didn't dawdle, and I think Thunder went with me, and we picked up some breakfast. Now I recall, what with the house being mostly done, Elmer wanted us to come out and begin breaking down the sun-dance arbor and cookshack and load them up.

When we got to the old place, Patti had worked herself into a terminal hissy fit. It was no later than early midmorning, but we got one accusation after another: "Look at you gettin' here so late. Lettin' that old man work down there by himself. Some warriors!" Actually, I walked in alone since Thunder had jumped out and gone on ahead down to the grounds. I must have looked so took aback, I was like a zombie, 'cause the next thing she said was, "Stop lookin' at me like that."

I began to defend myself, saying we were low on gas, and I'd only gone into town for an hour or so, but it was no use; her mind was made up. When I caught up with Thunder down at the sun-dance grounds, we both caught it all over again from Elmer. Pretty much the same line of talk, except he wasn't so nasty about it. He ended with another favorite saying of his: "I got my mind. I'm gon' be workin' over here. You two guys, you use you own minds, work over there."

Once we had our loads packed onto the back of the vehicles (we helped Elmer load his pickup, the difference of opinion notwithstanding), I commented to Thunder, "Patti must have put him up to it." To which he of course agreed, it was so obvious. I was really beginning to feel unappreciated by now and began a bit of a howl on the rankness and the ingratitude, until he cut me off, saying rather shortly that it was no different anywhere else.

Sadly, my subsequent time and experience have proven him mostly right. Patti's comment about the warrior had stung, though, and I'd somewhat disingenuously defended myself, saying, "I never claimed to be a warrior." But, like a few others who have perhaps not fit into their own culture too well, I did fantasize about being recognized and honored as a warrior for the people. Why else would I make all I could of the opportunity to live and work with a real, old-time, Lakota-speaking medicine man? I felt that this was my shot.

CHAPTER 6

Nebraska Mornings

ONCE AGAIN, I FIND I NEED TO BACKTRACK ON THIS RUN OF memories. Once the power was back on and I'd set up my camper in its little level spot in the woods at the bottom of the drive, the initial work was mostly bushwhacking and unloading the gear and tools each morning; I found myself with nearly two hours every day after sunrise to do what I liked. By this time, it was the beginning of late summer. The days were still quite hot, but parked where I was, in the shade of the north ridge, the afternoons and nights were quite comfortable. In the mornings, before Elmer and Pete came out, I would wander around the property, exploring the outbuildings and land. I particularly liked crossing the little creek and heading over to the pasture and the huge old barn. By this time in its life, the roof was fairly porous, but the interior had suffered little damage. Since it was built in the post-and-beam days, there were great big timbers everywhere, and the haymow was especially inviting. The old bale hoist and pulleys were still in their track under the roof, though the ropes were long gone, and the loft doors were impossible to shut. One had to get high above the floor of the mow, which was none too sturdy, onto a little walkway underneath the doors and, leaning out over empty air, reach the wooden handles on the insides—then try to pull them together to drop the inner swiveling bar into its catches. But the doors had either warped out of true or had been loosened on their hinges from years of banging around in the wind. I almost closed them a couple of times, but once when I tried it on a breezy morning and almost got pulled out, I had to give it up.

But from the haymow's elevated, south-facing vantage, I could look out over the endless Nebraska prairie, countless swells of earth rising and falling out of view. Outside the barn, there wasn't much to do in the old pasturage. There were a few cattle pens that were overgrown with marijuana, or *pegi* as it's called on the rez, and then the land quickly sloped off downhill to the west. To be up early on a summer morning and look out from such a place is a memory I think not many more will be able to have. There are so few of those old barns left.

One last little note, from about midway through my time there, during the rebuilding. From the very first, the place had a very deserted air about it. Elmer had commented, after the belated and burr-clogged visit from the Germans, that the spirits liked it there. Mother Earth had gone a long way, in thirty-odd years of vacancy, toward reclaiming herself. Once, again early in the morning, with no one else around, I'd gone out to the pasture across the creek. I'd gotten the strangest impression; I turned quickly to my left and seemed to glimpse a little man, very Indian-looking, seated on the top of a big old post that stuck up out of the ground. I mentioned it to Patti that evening when I went back to the old place to shower and eat. "Yeah, those little people are around us, just like you white people used to have." Or something like that.

I'd heard of the Pukwudgies from the time I'd spent back east among the Wampanoag; that was their name for the little folk. I'd also read of how they disliked the too-near presence of man and how most tribes were wary of them, not unlike the fairy faith in Celtic countries. Except for the Iroquois; the little folk managed to make friends there and even had a special dance the people danced for them. It shouldn't be too surprising; nearly every culture on earth has legends about a small, magically gifted race that inhabits remote areas. Anyone who has read the old stories of those who have claimed to have seen them can't help but question the commonplace denial: "There's no such thing." I've heard well-meaning white men say the same of the spirits, and I know that's wrong.

One other unrelated recollection is of something Elmer said, back at the old place, about the time of the visit from the horseback riders: "If bein' an Indian was easy, everybody'd be doin' it."

In a lot of ways, living and working on Indian time was far superior to doing so by the white man's regulated, eight-hour day. Instead of having to endure the monotony of going always to the same place and doing the same job with the same people five days a week, we did the work as it needed to be done. Admittedly, one of the things about Indian time that wasn't easy was the big schedule. Except for the occasional visits to the casino, there was no recreation or entertainment. No movie theater in Niobrara, no weekends off. Elmer had obviously had to work hard for most of his life, and there really wasn't any letting up. I remember several trips when driving the ten miles into town for a run to the hardware store seemed like a real treat. I also remember back at the old place, after dinner, I'd be inside watching TV with Pete and Patti, but Elmer would get up again before dark and be out in the yard or down at the sun-dance grounds. He'd go weeding, cleaning up the perimeter of the yard around the house. This being just inside rattlesnake country, it made sense to keep things trim.

By now, the upstairs rooms were finished, and a lot of Elmer
and Patti's clothing, blankets, and sun-dance paraphernalia
were going into winter storage up there. The heavy jackets were
coming out for work in the morning, and the frost lay heavily on
the ground by then. I recall driving on the new, upper driveway
one morning to call home on my cell phone, since coverage ceased
down in the draw between the ridges. I was wearing an old felt
slouch hat against the chill, and I was heading back down, when
here comes Elmer and Pete, heading in. They both started grinning when they saw me in that hat. It wasn't that bad looking,
only teasing one about one's hat, or anything outstanding about
one's appearance, is a favorite Indian thing. Elmer should talk. I
recall just before Dave Ross left, he and I were cleaning out the
tiny storage area in the ceremony house and the shed where old
sun-dance gear was kept, under Elmer's direction. We'd had
an early sweat, and there were piles of old prayer ties and flags
that hadn't been properly disposed of—that is, burned up in the
sweat-lodge fire after sweat. Dave and I were in the ceremony
house after dumping the first load and had just gotten back
inside, when here comes Elmer wearing a little baby sun hat with
the brim pulled down. It was all I could do to keep from holler-
ing, *"Gilligan!"* at him. So things were pretty easy between us
guys, but whenever Patti was around, things got really tense.

Thunder had taken off a little before the cold weather, after
having stayed and helped out for a few weeks. Unfortunately,
we never got to use the pressure washer he'd brought to prep
the outside of the house for repainting. Simply too much else to
do first. Time and finances were also against us; it would soon
be too cold to paint, even during the day—and the hundreds it
would cost for primer, paint, rollers, and more were out of reach.
Jamie, as I recall, had gotten himself a new job with the tribe,
so he wasn't around too much anymore, either. The last big job I
remember helping with was taking down a huge, old hackberry

tree that shaded the south side of the house and yard. I would have left it standing, but Elmer was concerned one of the limbs would come down on the roof in a storm, so it was out with the chainsaws. I had added to my stock of power tools during the summer and had also had to buy a new bar and chain for my chainsaw. It had slid out of the back of the pickup I was driving and come down on the tip, ruining it. Once the replacement parts were on, it worked just fine.

Unfortunately, after the tree was felled and the bigger limbs were cut up, I got it stuck trying to take down the trunk. Had to have Pete come and cut me loose. I had to wait awhile, since he was still cutting limbs, and he wasn't any too pleased when I promptly got in too deep again. "If I'd got my saw stuck, I wouldn't go back and cut into the same place," he grumbled at me. But we got it all down before dark, and I spent the next morning stacking firewood over by the new sweat lodges.

Most evenings, all through the summer, I'd head back to the old place with Pete and Elmer to have supper, then head out to be night watchman. Patti had charged me with keeping an eye on the old man more than once, and I'd try to be the last out most nights to do that. But once he realized what I was doing, he'd stop at the end of the gravel road and wave me past onto the highway. Although he had one glass eye and didn't see too good out of the other, he didn't like to be babysat.

But as he was still being occasionally called out of the area to do ceremony for folks, there were a very few days when I had the new place all to myself with very little work to do. Pete would stay and keep an eye on the old house, and I'd be where I was most of the time, anyway. By now, such amenities as the giant cable spool, which served as the main outdoor work surface, was at the new place, as well as the trash-burning barrel. One afternoon, Elmer had told me he and Patti would be away all the next day. He asked me to gather up all the trash, paper food wraps, and so on that had accumulated and burn it. For some reason, I took it into my head that I'd burn some of the plastic trash, as well. Some shingle wrappers, torn tarps, and miscellaneous. I didn't say a word about it, because I knew it was bad for the atmosphere. I guess I was so desperate for entertainment, I wanted a little of the bright light plastic makes when it burns. Just before he left, Elmer turned to me and said, "And don't burn no plastic." Busted again. That wasn't the only time I could tell he knew what I was thinking. The closer they are to being a full blood, and the closer they keep to their peoples' traditions, the more likely any Native person is to being telepathic. This was the most dramatic instance I can relate, and I know it seems impossible. But really it's only one of many measures by which one may gauge just how much modern technological society has lost to its members. I've heard it's the natural birthright of humanity. The aborigines of Australia call it "head-talk." The more "civilized" and farther from the earth a person's background is, the less likely he is to have any experience of it. Well, I haven't burned any plastic from that day to this.

That one day off was one of the most beautiful I remember of that whole time. This was early in the fall, sometime in September. I was done with the trash gathering and burning by about noon, and I had the little travel fridge in my camper stocked up, so I didn't have to leave the place for lunch or dinner. I recall I was on my way back from visiting the pear tree by late morning. A few yards east of where I was parked, on the opposite side of the drive, was an old carriage shed—or possibly it had housed some kind of horse-drawn farm machinery—but I'm thinking it was where the family had kept their good wagon or buggy. It was long, high, and narrower than any contemporary garage. Painted barn red, as were all the outbuildings, it had a nest of yellow jackets living in one of the walls. The pear tree stood a few feet west of it and was still bearing the yellow fruit, after none knew how many years. Just now they were coming ripe, so one had to be careful, as they were a source of attraction for the little wasps.

I think I'd gotten one or two little edible ones when I saw the snake. A thin, long-bodied, fast-moving serpent came out of the grass on the hillside, looked around like it was aching to kick some ass, and then headed off into the woods on the other side of the drive. I'd never seen a grayish-blue snake before. Later, when I told Pete about it, he said it was a blue racer, and I was lucky to have been well away from it when it emerged, as the species was highly aggressive, though not venomous. I'd also never before seen a snake that traveled so fast, keeping the upper ten or so inches of its body well above the ground. If things hadn't been so quiet that day, I'm sure it would never have shown itself.

It isn't easy to describe the sensation of peace and stillness that the memory of that afternoon recalls. We were some ten miles from the nearest highway, and the nearest neighbor was at least two miles away. This was before the opening of the hunting season, so there were no rifle shots; these came about a month later. The early afternoon sun lay aslant the long grasses, just turning golden by the side of the drive, and the shade beneath the cottonwoods along the creek bank was as deep blue as being underwater. No sound at all, except for the breeze sliding around the ridge now and again and setting the cottonwood leaves to talking. These will stir in the slightest breath of wind, and even they were mostly still that day. The sky was an enormity of blue overhead, and after seeing the snake, absolutely nothing happened the rest of the day. It was great.

But back again to November, and the way things were after the blowup and scoldings was not good. It was just before the weather became truly cold that I began to experience the symptoms of hypertension, and the sinusitis that had begun that summer was getting worse and draining my energy. I'm afraid my memories of that time are somewhat clouded. I seem to recall

Patti's lighting into me again, this time because I'd mentioned that I was feeling unwell. She'd yelled, "We can't have sick folks around!" So I never brought it up to Elmer, and I very much doubt she did. It seemed he was no abler to defend me against that woman than I was able to defend him. All I can say is, when a scene you're committed to because you believe in it turns ugly, it really is dispiriting.

The temperature was falling below freezing every night now, and the skies in the day were a stark, November gray. There were almost no visitors or casual volunteers anymore, just the four of us. I remember one trip with Pete into Niobrara when it was practically a winter afternoon. We'd gone to get the large propane tank that fed the kitchen range filled and take it back to the new house. That was the trip he told me of his days as a mechanic and a pipe carver in a shop. I recall I was glad to get away from the place. Patti was there more and more, arranging the furniture, setting up the kitchen, and giving orders. No manners, no asking for anything, just telling us off. I remember how I'd resented not being able to listen to *A Prairie Home Companion* on Saturday evenings when I was married. Now the new season of the show was about to start, and here I was in exactly the same kind of dysfunctional situation. I remember that evening of the first broadcast; I simply stayed in the cab of my camper and listened as long as I could before I had to go help pitch firewood into the basement through an empty window so we could fire up the old furnace.

Speaking of which, the long drive I made to buy the two sizes and several lengths of stovepipe to get the old octopus furnace fireable again was a lot of fun. I had to drive north across some forty miles of Nebraskan tundra to a little town on the border between North Dakota and South Dakota. Can't recall the town or the name of the hardware place, but it was more of an emporium than a mere store. They were known to have all kinds of odd sizes of nearly everything, really, and they had what I needed.

The old pipe had rusted away over the decades, but the furnace itself was still good to go. I remember I had to use an adapter to go from a seven- to an eight-inch diameter, fit and secure an elbow, and clean out the coal dust and compacted ash from the bottom of the chimney. Then I drilled starter holes all along the seams and used sheet-metal screws to fasten it all together. Coming back from town on another run and seeing the blue woodsmoke coming from the chimney gave me a good feeling.

One funny thing, though. I had let my hair grow long for years before I ever came to Santee, and I must have looked quite the hippie. Or at least I did to the rabid Reaganite at the emporium. I'd had to go upstairs to the clerk's offices to get a purchase order in order to go out to the supply shed. This one guy at the very back of the room had his desk front covered with pictures of Ronnie R., plus little tiny flags on top. When he saw me come in, he started as if he'd seen a ghost. Like my appearance had hit him in his flight-or-fight plexus. The look on his face fairly screamed, "My God! A hippie! I thought Boss Reagan ran 'em all out of the country."

By the time that trip was done and the old furnace was piped into the chimney, winter had set in. It was a race to clear out all the rest of the furniture and gear from the old house and set it up in the new. I had at some point announced my intention to leave and visit my family over the holidays. It seemed as if everyone was buttoning their lips and trying to finish the work with a minimum of friction. Relations were strained, and there wasn't much joking anymore. Thunder had left soon after the morning Elmer had gotten after us. There was one funny incident, though. A lot of Indian men will, when they wish to indicate direction, point with their lips. The indication is clear when they do it, but when I tried it, Pete just burst out laughing, and even Elmer had to grin.

The morning I left was two days before Thanksgiving that year. Elmer and Pete were gone to the old house, bringing back the kitchen range. I told Patti good-bye and shook her hand, trying to leave in a good way. I unplugged my camper and made sure everything inside was lashed down and rolled down and locked the rear panel door. On the way out, going through a wooded part of the road, I passed Elmer and Pete coming back. I waved, but neither waved back. Despite everything I'd done over the year, and despite the impossible conditions, I still felt like I was letting the old man down. But I had helped them through a difficult transition, had mostly a good time doing it, and I was leaving with a "my work here is done" feeling.

I had either been sufficiently unwise or creative enough to have installed a tiny woodstove in the box of the furniture van I'd converted into my camper. I'd been using it, those cold nights, enough to have creosote stains below where the stovepipe exited. The wind from going down the road also blew some (cold) ashes into the living space. I remember I stopped at a little convenience store for gas, and a couple of Santee guys came along and couldn't believe I had a stove in there.

"Does it work?" one of them asked.

"Well, it's kept me warm at night so far."

That holiday season, I lived in my camper. First in one married sister's driveway, then another's. I was looking for a place to rent, since I'd decided not to go on living with Elmer and Patti. In fact, I was so burned out after one year that I didn't get back for ceremony 'til late spring. By then, I'd found a little rental home in a small town south of Omaha, whose landlord allowed me to keep my little dog. During early November, I'd been in town and seen a flyer for a breeder of shih tzus. I'd been really taken with this sturdy toy breed when my ex and I'd rescued one that had been abandoned. That breeder was the first place I stopped after leaving the rez. I picked out a black, eight-week-old female, and we camped for a night at Niobrara State Park. That day, I named her Belle.

It being late November, Belle and I had the campground all to ourselves. We had a good time getting to know each other, and even though she growled at me once that first day, we've gotten pretty close over the intervening twelve years. We've moved once but have lived in the same small town. She's had a couple of pals adopted from the shelter, also shih tzus. She's had one litter of puppies, and her daughter Lizzie and mate, Buddy, are with us now, along with the little gray-and-white cat I got as a kitten from my first neighbor in Louisville.

I moved with Belle into the little rental house the day before the winter solstice in 1999. That was a very peaceful winter, apart from reliving Patti's (and my ex's) abusive behavior. I didn't get into the *pegi* I'd brought until a month or so later. I'd found a little Chinese-style opium pipe at a local antique shop, though I had qualms about using any pipe other than my *canunpa*. Nonetheless, one gray day in late February, I snuck into the little rear room where I'd squirreled it away, bagged up a little of it, got the pipe out, and just as I was putting one into the other, I happened to look out the east window—and what should I see but a great big owl in the pin oak tree, staring right at me. That was not the first time one of the night flyers had come to me since I'd started praying to Grandfather, and each time, it had presaged a death, or at least a serious misfortune. I stupidly went ahead and smoked it, even knowing what I did.

Chapter 7

Sweating at Patti's

A FEW WEEKS LATER, I GOT WORD THAT ONE OF MY COUSINS had died of a heart attack. Confusion set in, and I became so conflicted over it that I threw out all the smoking stuff I had and kept on making my monthly ceremony ties. I didn't keep in touch with Elmer and Patti at all. I really needed a break.

And so when winter had departed and spring was well under way, I left Belle and the cat in the care of my neighbors and headed back to Santee. Imagine my surprise to find Elmer gone and Patti in the midst of selling off as much of his gear and equipment as she could in a yard sale. Pete was still there, and he told me Elmer had gone back to Rosebud about midwinter. He couldn't say too much more, with Patti there. Her version of events was that he'd gotten a sudden need to go back among his relatives of the Sicangu Lakota. He'd just taken his pipe, gotten into his pickup, and driven back to South Dakota by himself. Later on, I learned from Pete that Patti had continued her abusive, loud-mouthed treatment of the menfolk. Pete himself was being more or less held hostage by her refusal to pay him anything or even to prepare more than one meal a day. It goes without saying that she had maintained control over the resources of the household. Pete also told me that just before Elmer left, she had gone into town one afternoon, and her parting shot had been, "And don't just sit around here all day talkin' about old drunk times."

Pete said he wasn't going to tell me everything Elmer had said about her except, "That's a greedy woman." Such a person would not be fit to hold the *canunpa* of a *wicasa wakan*. I also noticed that Waziya and Tegi were looking skinny as hell, and the little yellow cur had gone altogether. When I asked Patti about it, she just mumbled some excuse about them not being well. I should have realized they were starving. When Waziya saw me coming, she ran to me as to a savior, and even tough guy Tegi tried to grin at me. It was funny for a moment: Ever see a perpetually scowling tough guy suddenly try to look friendly? Like his face was way out of practice for it? That's just how he looked. If I hadn't been so preoccupied with Elmer's absence, I would have thought to go to town and buy a big bag of dog chow. The next time I went there, they were both gone.

Anyhow, there were a bunch of folks at the yard sale, mostly white ranchers and guys from town. I got a few things, even buying back the generator I'd gotten when Elmer's had been stolen. The way Patti told it, she had talked to him over the phone and invited him to come and get his stuff, but he wouldn't come. Again, I should have known better, but I listened to her spin her yarn and got all sympathetic. I found out later that year, having tracked down Elmer on my own, that she'd told him to come alone, and the spirits had told him not to go.

Going with her into the house, Patti showed me how she'd wrapped the stem of her *canunpa* with prayer ties and said the spirits had told her it was time for her to be leading ceremony, and not just for the women but as a medicine woman. At that time, I didn't know better, but such a creature doesn't exist within Lakota culture. But I didn't know, and for a while, I took her at her word.

The following month, I attended one of her sweats. We two were about the only ones in the lodge, as I recall, and it was kind of freaky. She asked me for a sun-dance song, and fortunately by that time I had at least one memorized. She sang the songs to the four directions, the sweat-lodge stones, and calling in the spirits, but there was nothing happening in the ceremony house afterward. I found out later it had been emptied of all the beautiful ceremonial implements Elmer had been given or acquired, as well as most of what little furniture it had had. Those, too, had disappeared, but the worst was when she began quizzing me about how I'd gotten my pipe. I told her the truth, that my ex had given it to me just before my first sun dance so that I could help pray for the healing of a little baby Indian girl who had spina bifida and fluid on the brain. Her father was a Kiowa, a Vietnam vet who'd been exposed to Agent Orange.

Well, she managed to get around me with her line of talk, convinced me that that hadn't been the right way to get a pipe. The fact that the prayers had been answered didn't seem to interest her. Long story short, she ended up convincing me to put my pipe up on the hill. That was an evil deed, and a misguided one on my part, and I know she has since paid for it, as well as for her abuse of Elmer, and paid hard.

PART 3
Rosebud, 2000–01

CHAPTER 8

Hau-hau-hau!

ORTUNATELY, I GUESS, ON SOME LEVEL, PATTI'S STORY
wasn't adding up for me. She still wouldn't tell me where
Elmer was exactly, and I had a growing desire to see and talk
to the old man. He was the sun-dance chief, after all, not her.
So, one day just after sun dance, I used long-distance directory
assistance to track the old man down. Turns out, he was staying
with one of his sons, Norman, which was who I ended up talking
to and getting directions from. When I once again left the animals
at home in the care of a neighbor and got to the Rosebud rez for
the first time, they were just fixing to sweat at Norman's. Also,
Elmer, who was seated at a bench by the door of the lodge, greeted me with the traditional greeting between two males: "Hau-
hauhau!" We shook hands, he had a big grin, and Norman asked
me if I wanted to sweat.

I told him not after my long drive; I'd wait 'til the weekend,
which was the monthly ceremony. Later on, Norman remarked to
me, "Dad was sure glad to see you." It was pretty nice to be made
so welcome.

Later on, Elmer and I got to talking. It seems Patti hadn't been
quite truthful to me, and she had demanded that he come alone.
It was a weird request, because there was no way that old man

could have loaded all his tools, gear, sun-dance appurtenances, and tipis by himself. Or at least, what there was left of them. I told him about the yard sale and about Patti starting to run sweat and ceremony herself. I also told him about buying the generator; I promised to return it to him on my next visit. He got a sort of funny, almost embarrassed look and sort of mumbled his thanks. Later on, I mentioned this to Nico, who'd come up for ceremony. "It was like he knew I'd bought it," I said.

"He knew," Nico replied. We didn't discuss how he'd known; we knew how.

Elmer was living in an old mobile home donated by the tribe. There was no ceremony house, so after sweat, we had to move all the furniture into the hall and tape blankets over all the windows and the mirror, which covered a section of one wall. There was also a young lady named Maidcha from Germany staying there to hang out with the *wicasa wakan* and doing some work around the place. She wasn't one of the regular Germans, I learned. Her father had come over for a doctoring for his cancer. Maidcha was good to have around; she was a good cook, although a bit chatty. This ceremony was actually her father's *wopila*, or thanksgiving for the doctoring. He got through it and the next day presented Elmer with an envelope. I happened to see Elmer peek into it. I couldn't tell how many hundreds were in there, but I do know it was a voluntary payment. Elmer never charged.

So here I was having missed my fourth year, without a *canunpa*, all due to Patti's efforts to win me over to her side. I recall that Elmer's take on Patti was, "There's something wrong with her mind. And I'm not gon' say one more thing 'bout her."

Before we got to that point, I'd told him about Patti's claim to have been called by the spirits to do ceremony. Elmer said, "I know 'bout that. It's not regular earth spirits she's callin' in it, it's . . . I don't know right word." He paused, searching for the right word in English. "I don't know what to call 'em."

"Is it evil spirits?" I asked, somewhat concerned.

"No. It's—I don't know how to say it."

I recall there was some consternation among the family members and sun dancers at my having attended Patti's little sideshow. All I could do was plead innocence: I simply hadn't known where else to turn.

It was hot up in South Dakota that summer, and the flies were bad. There was a big tear in the screen door on Elmer's double-wide, and after a week of buying that awful flypaper, I finally broke down and went to town, got some screening, and went to work on reinstalling it. I finally got the panel off, removed the keeper that held the screen in, and was wrestling it into place when Maidcha came along and said, "That's a good thing you're doing, Karl." It was the same thing an older Lakota woman had said to me back at the new place, in Santee. One afternoon, she came to visit Elmer and Patti and to see the new digs. It was early on, and I was in the process of taking down a volunteer elm sapling from the yard and cutting it up. Just having at it with the chainsaw, kind of showing off.

Norman and his wife, Shannon, had a big room on its own foundation on the south side of their trailer. It had a couch, a table and chairs, a big color TV, and lots of cushions for seating during the feast after ceremony. It also had good air conditioning, so some evenings we'd end up there. It was at one evening meal there that Elmer got to instructing me how to eat properly. After taking a small bit of the various foods and placing some on the spirit plate to be taken outside as an offering afterward, he told me, "Say, 'Mitakuye Oyasin'" (all my relations). Then you could eat. Of course, we'd been feeding the spirits at mealtime since Santee, but this was the other important bit.

Finally, the talk turned to retrieving Elmer's sun-dance gear, tools, and clothes from Santee. I remember having a few feelings of frustration, after having worked so hard and so long under such aggravating conditions to lick that old farmhouse into shape, only to have him leave and end up in a mobile home. But that was his choice, and I could see his adherence to Lakota tradition in his decision. According to tribal custom, as far as I understand it, the woman owns the home and has the say on what happens therein. Of course, that doesn't give her the right to her (ex-) man's things. She's supposed to leave them outside, in case he decides to go or if she gets fed up and tells him to.

I had to leave and get back home, but at next month's ceremony—September, I believe—we began discussing it in earnest. One good thing had come out of my keeping up with Patti: I knew her schedule. God knows what she'd told them about herself and the old man, but the last thing she'd said to me after her August ceremony was that she'd be flying over to Germany to run ceremony and would be gone for a certain stretch of time. I remember stopping in at the new place on my way back from Rosebud and finding it deserted. No dogs, no Patti, no Pete. But hanging just inside the door of the old shop was Elmer's eagle-wing fan that he always used in sweat and his little buckskin bag of herbs he sprinkled onto the grandfathers as they came in. I figured Patti was gone overseas and wouldn't miss it. I managed to get these things back to him on my own, and after ceremony, we started getting ready to go back for the rest of it.

Gonna break the narrative here. In case you're starting to think this mostly *wasicu* guy's really getting in over his head, you're right. I've since been told that around the altar of nearly every traditional *wicasa wakan*, this kind of weird spiritual politics and infighting goes on. This is why so few people were able to really spend a long time with Elmer. It just burns you out to be in the midst of all that, being pulled and pressured to side with this faction or that, and enduring slights and worse for all your trouble.

All this notwithstanding, once I'd told Elmer that Patti would be off doing her bogus ceremony in Germany, he was ready to go and get the stuff. We decided to leave early in the morning. This must have been just after the new moon in September of 2000.

CHAPTER 9

Reclaiming Elmer's Stuff

THE NIGHTS WERE STARTING TO GET COOL AGAIN, AND I RE-
call we all got up early, before first light. While Elmer was
on his second cup of coffee, Maidcha called his attention to a big,
white spider that was building a web inside the window next
to his easy chair. It had only six legs, and we speculated on this
being a good sign for our trip. Elmer said, "If you ever need to get
the spiders outta you' house, just tell 'em. They know! Iktomi's
got a spirit. But them flies, they don't."

There was a young man with us, Indian Bill from Whitefish,
who'd come for ceremony and who said he'd help out. So with
Maidcha tending the home fires, we three set off in my pickup, it
being the biggest vehicle available. Before we even got to Mission,
though, we had a flat tire. We pulled into the big service station
and convenience store on the edge of town. Bill got out to look at
it and found a piece of iron I'd driven over. I was able to fix the
flat with a can of Fix-A-Flat, then I gassed 'er up, and we were
on our way.

I recall the day as being cloudy, mostly overcast. The day
slowly grew light enough to see by as we approached the wet-
lands that border the Missouri River as it flows west along the
Nebraska–South Dakota line—well, the river is the border. Bill

and Elmer were conversing at intervals, sometimes in English, sometimes in Lakota. At one point, we crossed a little bridge over a nondescript body of water in a marshy section, with the body of a fresh-killed mallard lying by the side of the road. "Hey," said Bill to Elmer. "You want to stop and get that duck fur?"

"No," said Elmer. "Just keep goin'."

When I asked Bill what he wanted it for, he told me the shiny, iridescent bands on the neck were sometimes used for decorations on pipe stems.

The day and the journey wore on. It must have been a little before noon when we crossed the big bridge into Nebraska. At that point, we were only a short drive from Niobrara and Santee. The atmosphere in the truck began to get tense. We all knew that the old man had a right to his own things. Nevertheless, we were about to commit criminal trespass, and breaking and entering, and probably, according to Patti, grand larceny.

We got into and then through Niobrara and made the turnoff for Santee. This time, it was weird going down those roads with Elmer, even though I'd traveled them so many times before. Now we were here with a grab-and-git attitude. As we turned off the county highway onto the gravel and past the little stone bridge that crossed the creek that eventually joined the little stream between the house and barn, I saw a buzzard sitting in a tree. Just as we passed under, it flew off to the left across our path. A feeling came over me with this sign that we would do all right; that we'd get the stuff back and get free and clear. I recall we stopped at the nearest farmhouse, at Elmer's direction. He got out to check with the fella who lived there. We all trooped in and had coffee and a smoke, sat around while he and Elmer conferred. He said that yes, Patti was gone. This guy was an unknown to me, but Elmer knew him well—well enough that when he learned of the reason for our visit, he agreed to park up on the gravel road where the drive joined it and honk if anybody showed up. He agreed that Patti holding on to Elmer's possessions wasn't right. Elmer agreed to the plan, and we were off.

Things were really tense as we made our way up the gravel road to the hillcrest where the upper and lower drives began. We turned down the lower drive, between the two ridges. When we got down to the farmyard, the place was deserted. It had regained some of its *Blair Witch* ambience. Some big limbs from one of the cottonwoods had come down and were lying where they'd fallen. Somehow the air of disarray combined with the day's mood to lend an ominous, even threatening, aspect. Before, even on the most unharmonious occasions, the little valley had always had a peaceful, serene atmosphere, but not anymore. I don't know if it was due to Patti's weird ceremonies or Elmer's abandonment, but it didn't feel as if the spirits liked it there anymore.

We pulled up and came to a stop. Waited a moment. No sign of anyone. None of the dogs showed up, of course. I'd told Elmer that it was no matter if the house was locked, because I knew of a basement window, the one I'd pitched firewood through the previous winter, that was closed only by piece of board that was just set into the frame. So I was the first in, through the window into the basement, then upstairs to open the door. They were both waiting for me on the back step. It was kinda funny how they both looked surprised when I opened up. But in we went, not much was said, and we all headed upstairs, where Elmer's clothes, drum, and sun-dance gear were. We never touched anything that was Patti's. Well, almost nothing. We got a lot of mud on the new carpet and didn't exactly take time to clean it up.

As one might expect, the next hours or so are kind of a blur. All I can recall from getting Elmer's things out of the upstairs is that once, between loads, Bill and I came upon two bald eagle feathers. Bill asked Elmer something about them in Lakota, holding them up. Elmer replied, "No, but take 'em; they're good feathers."

We found the buffalo robes, the sun-dance drum, Elmer's eagle-feather war bonnets, and a lot of other ceremonial gear. As Bill remarked to me, "I'd give my left nut for this stuff." I sort of kept the two feathers separate. I had an idea that what Bill and I were doing might rate the distinction of a warrior, and I found out later that he felt the same.

Once we'd loaded the stuff from the house into the rear seat of my pickup, we divided our efforts. Elmer sent me off to the old machine shop down by the sweat lodges and asked Bill to help him get into the garage, which was much closer to the house. I saw Bill pick up and swing one of those heavy main drive shafts from the interior of a transmission against the padlock on the garage door. Those things are mean. I didn't hear too many impacts before they stopped.

By then, I was at the doorway to the shed. I began taking out all the hand tools, pitchforks, shovels, digging bar, and so on. At some point, Elmer came down and told me to hurry up, so I started carrying the tools up to the truck. He and Bill were still transferring things out of the garage, so we had to work together to pack the pickup's bed to hold as much as it could.

By now, things were getting into the mad scramble, "let's get the hell out of here" phase. We'd been there for over an hour, and the sense of "it's time to go" was becoming insistent. I think we all felt it increase the longer we stayed. I remember the last item we got back was the heavy log splitter—the massive kind on wheels with a tow hitch, about eight feet long. It was parked behind one of the smaller sheds between the house and the drive, and Elmer was damned if he was gonna leave it. It had been a gift to him and, at first, when Bill and I refused to move it as he asked, he got mad, bent over, and made to pick up the hitch end by himself. We frantically explained ourselves: "No, Elmer. We'll take it, but we gotta back the truck up to it and hitch it on." Thankfully, he listened and realized this would of course be much faster and easier, not to say possible.

That's what we did, and we were at last ready to leave. For some reason, probably because the lower drive we'd come in on was muddy, I took the steeper upper drive out. I recall setting the traction on 4WL, downshifting into second, and having to give it a lot of gas just to get up that first steep climb. As we passed over the one stretch of bare rock, the rear wheels lost traction, and I shifted all the way down into first, muttering, "Don't spin it. Don't spin it." Then I shut up and got us out of there.

Our lookout had disappeared by the time we hit the gravel road, but we didn't take the route out that would have led past his place. Instead, I took us by the much emptier back way. There were only two widely separated farmhouses to pass, one of which was so well screened by ancient cottonwoods that any passing vehicle would be known only by its noise and dust. It also led us to a section of the highway that allowed us to get across the Chief Standing Bear Memorial Bridge into South Dakota without going through Niobrara. The Department of the Army, which had charge of Indian affairs and reservations before the formation of the Bureau of Indian Affairs, had in its military wisdom settled the Isanti Nakota—after the rising in Minnesota in 1862—on land that had already been reserved for the Ponca. I recalled Patti saying that the two tribes usually got along, but whenever there was any friction, the Ponca never failed to throw this in the Santee's teeth.

Once we were well away, our mood turned celebratory. I had a little bag of candy of some kind, and after I'd popped one, Elmer asked me, "Izzat candy?"

"Yeah," I said, offering him the bag. He shared back to Bill, and I recalled that there were some dances, usually held at pow-wows, that concluded with hard candy being thrown about and distributed to the public, mostly to the kids. This seemed like one of those kinds of times. We sure weren't going to toast our success. We were quietly jubilant. And hungry!

After we'd gotten safely across the river into South Dakota, in a little under an hour, we stopped for a late breakfast at a highway diner. There was a fairly full parking lot, plus several semis, so we thought the food was probably good there—but we had to park way off in a back row. Elmer was looking a little frazzled by the aftereffects of all the adrenaline. We'd all been fairly high on it during our "heist." Bill and I went inside and ordered one of the biggest breakfasts ever, after I'd taken Elmer's travel mug inside for a coffee refill. Taking it back out to him, I asked him again if he wanted to eat, but he said, "No, it's all right. You guys go on. I just gon' stay here."

I figured he knew himself best, so I went back in and finished my steak and eggs and bacon and hash browns with a short stack and coffee. We came back out, hit the road, and by early evening, we were back in Rosebud.

I don't recall if it was that evening or a few days later that we had a sweat to pray and give thanks for our successful trip. At some point earlier in the day, as we were unloading the last of the things, I'd approached Elmer concerning the matter of the two feathers. After we'd gotten most of it stowed to his satisfaction, he sat down in his easy chair, and I waited a bit and then asked him, "Elmer, if you're OK with it, Bill and I would like to have those two eagle feathers we took back."

He didn't say anything at first, just stared at me kind of sternly, but then he just said, "All right," in that quiet voice of his. I had the feeling he didn't actually approve of our request, since one is supposed to wait until one is given such a mark of accomplishment. But he didn't think we didn't deserve them. In one way, it was a very big deal to ask for them; in another, it really wasn't much considering what we'd done and risked for him—and, by extension, for the people. Because that was the nature of doing anything for a traditional medicine man: Anything good that came to him, he'd either pass on or he'd use it to further his life's work, which was to help and pray for his people and for all living things—even those of his people, as I'd seen in Santee and was to see again, who were giving him a hard time.

Before the sweat, I was the fire keeper once again. About halfway through the burn, Bill came up to where I was sitting, and we talked for a while. I gave him the feather with the beadwork on it, and after a little while, he gave me a little fluff of eagle down, "breath feathers," since they stir at the slightest breath. Just about then, I looked up and noticed the wind had carried an ember or spark onto the loose bark and sticks next to the woodpile and started a blaze. It was small and no trouble to extinguish, and after I'd done so, we shook hands on our exchange, and he went back to the trailer.

But just before the sweat, we were joined by Florian Bluethunder, the same one who had the bag of sandwiches ripped out of his hand by a starving Waziya back in Santee. Elmer led us off, after the first rounds of songs, by thanking the spirits for "helpin' us get them things back. Been prayin' 'bout that for quite a while, but them boys came in and did it. Now we back home."

Florian prayed too, a long prayer in Lakota, and I couldn't make much out of it, except he seemed to be commending Bill and myself to the spirits for helping Elmer, since I caught the phrase *wasicu takoja*, or white (man) grandson, and boy, that was plenty gratifying!

I find that I've forgotten to mention that at one of the monthly ceremonies held at the new place in Santee, I'd gone in for a doctoring. I recall this because afterward, or rather, during the last part of the ceremony, just before the lights came back on, the spirits had gifted me with the ceremony flags. This means that after the doctorings were over, after the thanksgiving song had been sung, the spirits would pull the yard-long strips of varicolored cloth off the flagpoles, which were saplings stuck in earth in coffee cans, and would throw them in a ball into the lap of whomever they'd chosen that night. Sometimes nobody got them, and they'd be burned in the sweat fire. The tobacco that was bundled into the uppermost corner of each flag was cut out, still in its cloth, and this would go into the fire, but the cloths would be kept and reused for prayer ties.

CHAPTER 10

Sweating with the Relatives

I NOW RECALL MY DOCTORING WASN'T AT EITHER PLACE IN Nebraska but at monthly ceremony in Rosebud. I had received the flags at the last ceremony I attended in Santee, but I find the more I struggle to recall these events correctly, the more comes back, but not always before I've already recounted events that took place later. And so, my doctoring wasn't at Elmer's when he had his trailer set up at Norman's, but earlier, when he had moved it onto his old property at Ironwood Hilltop.

A family of his close relations, headed by one Irene, had taken up residence in the house Elmer and his first wife and kids had lived in, and they were none too pleased to have the old man back. I can't recall all the arrangements as well as I could for Santee, but the first time I sweated in South Dakota, the lodge was set up on the edge of a steep bank, running down quite a distance to a creek bottom. Several of Elmer's sons were present, including Johnson.

The sweat seemed to go all right, until the end. Elmer had lasted all the way through but had been feeling sicker and sicker as the rite proceeded. This was because Johnson had come in drunk, and the spirits were taking it out on the old man. When we all crawled out to shake hands and get dressed, Elmer started tottering off balance. He began to stagger out of control downhill and would surely have plunged over the bank if I hadn't caught him. After I'd gotten him back uphill and we sat down to dry off and dress, I lit a cigarette. Johnson came by, all unheeding, and asked me for a drag in mime. What does he proceed to do but walk off with the whole butt, without even a *pilamaye*. Later on, I saw him more or less forcibly detained in the old house by the rest of the family, who were sageing him off. He looked angry, but the rest of the folks seemed to be looking daggers at me and the other attendees. It seemed Irene and her bunch liked to play at ceremony and spiritual commitment but still liked to party. They made things pretty rough for the old man until he finally did move to Norman and Shannon's a few miles up the road.

Well, that was enough for one visit. I went back to my little rental home in Nebraska and my little dog Belle, who had been cared for by my new next-door neighbors. Belle loved to jump in the truck and go riding with Dad—and it was on a grocery run into Omaha with Belle the next week that I got a call on my cell phone from Patti.

I should probably explain at this point that I had done something that, in hindsight, was very stupid. On the trip to Santee when I'd picked up the fan and bag of herbs, I'd foolishly left a note for her asking her to return Elmer's things to him. So naive. There are other stupid things I'd said or done during my time with Elmer, but they weren't essential to the narrative, so I've very thoughtfully left them out. This, I can't. I'd left the note, then gone on to instigate the retrieval mission. So she knew who to call. "Where are you?" was her first demand. "Are you up at Rosebud?"

"No, Patti. I'm in Omaha." There followed a brief but spirited back-and-forth, in which I may have admitted to being involved. But the last thing I said to her was, "Patti, you wouldn't tell me where he was when I asked you, and because of that, I missed my fourth year sun dancing; that's all I have to say." I knew it wasn't proper, in the Lakota tradition, to bicker it up to the point of it becoming an "argument," let alone lighting into her like I wanted, so I held my tongue and hung up. But of course that wasn't the end of it.

Well, a week or so later, I got a call from my dad. It seems Patti had called him and threatened to call the state police and have me arrested unless he paid her a fairly hefty sum in damages. I found out later he'd actually gone up there and paid her in person the amount she'd requested. At the moment, though, he was only interested in giving me a hard time. First, he asked me if I'd actually been involved, and when I said yes, he asked me what I'd been thinking—and as soon as I began to explain, he cut me off, telling me he didn't care who had whose things, it was wrong to go around breaking into people's homes, and so on, blah blah. He was really enjoying lighting into me, as he always had, after a pretense at a fair inquiry. First he asks for my side of the story, then he won't listen to it. But after a thorough parent-to-child chewing-out, he let out his kicker and said, "I don't think Elmer's leading you in a good way." His timing and the way he said it told me he'd been long awaiting such an opportunity. Despite being offended, I decided not to tell him the whole thing had been my idea. I could sense over the phone, just by the so-superior tone in his voice, his immense gratification at being able to dump on something that mattered to me.

But what of that? Another memory bubble has surfaced, which is that after we'd returned the gear and tools, and after the sweat, I'd spent a few days at Elmer's, long enough to attend a celebration thrown by some of the local sun dancers and Gilli to mark the return of it all. Bill had taken off for home soon after the sweat. The next weekend, a bunch of folks showed up to help throw a celebratory feast.

I recall that Gilli came in with several young men and a
drum, and they set up in the kitchen of Elmer's mobile home.
Before they could get started, though, Elmer vehemently, almost
angrily, forbade Gilli from singing any of the newfangled songs
he'd come up with. They started out and went through several
songs that sounded all right, but even though I couldn't make
out the words, when he disobeyed his dad and sang one or two
not from the traditional canon, I could tell. They sounded wrong
somehow. Elmer looked up from his seat in the living room with
an expression of displeasure but said nothing. I guess that's why
Gilli had all young men with him. They didn't know better or
didn't care like most old-timers would.

Earlier, Gilli had sort of made a casual attempt to impress me
with his spiritual credentials, speaking of songs he'd learned and
"songs that have come through me," but I wasn't buying any.
He asked me a little later, when the women had come and were
laying out a big feed, if I had an Indian name, as they wished to
honor me for my part in our escapade, but I told him I didn't.
That wasn't quite true, but I didn't feel good about revealing such
a thing to someone like him. Later still, Lorna, one of the women
leaders, called me a hero. That was all right. First time I'd been
called that.

Looking back again, I believe I was right the first time: Elmer
had gone to live first at Norman and Shannon's. A little later,
when the tribe had gotten him his old double-wide, he'd had it
set up on his old property at Ironwood. It was from here that he
ran his ceremonies and to and from which we left to retrieve his
things from Patti. Later, he had to move back to Norman's—and
later still to a new location a mile or two from Ironwood, due to
persecution and being taken advantage of by the family, which
was why he'd left Rosebud and gone to Santee back in the late
1980s. I recall that when I first got back together with him at
Norman's, he was very affable and asked me where I was living,

in the town or country? I told him, "In a little town about twenty miles south of Omaha."

"Where in town?" he asked me. "East side? West side?"

"Little house I'm renting on the east side."

"Oh," he said.

On my next visit, but before we took our run to Santee, he remarked on the weight I'd gained, in a not-too-pleased voice. "'Nough for two guys," he grumbled.

This after, on my bending down to enter the *inipi*, one of the young Lakota guys had giggled and said, 'He blocks out the light."

This was of course before the first seven rocks came in, during which time silence is observed. My chocaholism, coupled with the enervating effects of the sinusitis I'd been suffering from, had led to a long period of inactivity. That plus living in town meant there wasn't the constant, hard, physical labor of living way out on the rez.

But getting back to that first summer, after we'd gotten the things back and had our celebration, I'd gone in for a doctoring for my sinuses. I was sitting on the floor of the living room of the double-wide, making a set of flags and ties for my *wopila*. In most cases, the healing isn't fully accomplished until the thank-you part of the ceremony is completed. I was sitting there making my ties, talking a little with Maidcha, the German girl, when the most extraordinary feeling came over me. I could feel my sinuses becoming less painful and inflamed with nearly every prayer tie that left my fingers. The more I did, the better they felt.

By now, fall was getting on once again, and I began to spend more time away from Rosebud, except I'd go up once a month at the new moon for ceremony. It was easier knowing someone was with Elmer while I was away, at first Maidcha and then one or another of his relatives. The stories I'd heard about nearly all his boys being drunks who'd steal from the old man sort of receded from my mind since Norman was around a lot, and he seemed to be keeping the rest in line. At first.

I recall making two such trips, one in October and one in November, when I was hauling up a quite a few supplies. I'd stop at the Surplus Warehouse in Wahoo and load up on canned goods and items useful to the old man. Then I'd make the long drive north to O'Neill, then west through the Nebraska outback to Valentine and on into South Dakota. On both of these trips, as soon as I crossed the Mission, South Dakota, city limits, an oncoming vehicle full of Native passengers would pass, and the driver would give me the clenched-fist salute. From my generation, that meant, "Power to the people." I used to wonder how they knew it was me, as I didn't know many folks there, or whether it was the spirit moving the driver at that moment.

It must have been during the October trip that Elmer and I had our first road trip. Elmer asked me to drive him over to Pipestone, Minnesota, in the heart of the Dakota/Nakota/Lakota homeland. As a pipe carver and an enrolled tribal member, Elmer was entitled to go up to the quarry and take away as much of the sacred stone as he desired, with no charge levied by the National Park Service, which now administers the site. I have heard and read of many Native people saying that this is the only spot in the world where this particular type of stone is found. I've also heard that there is another deposit of catlinite somewhere in rural China. I realize that "somewhere in China" covers a lot of ground, but that's what I've heard.

We set off early on a Saturday morning. As we pulled onto the highway, I turned the radio to the South Dakota Public Radio channel. I was and still am a fan of the program Car Talk, and it was going to be a long drive. After a while, the show came on, and one of the first callers described a problem with his European-made vehicle—a Volkswagen or Peugeot, I think. Elmer and I listened carefully as the show hosts, Tom and Ray, painstakingly described what they thought was ailing the thing and how to track down the specific component responsible. It was something to do with the car's air-intake system, and they recommended that as soon as the caller found a small canister containing charcoal pellets (or some such) for purifying exhaust gases for warming the carburetor, he should take it off and throw it away. The brusque delivery of this last line cracked us both up. Tom and Ray went into their trademark cackling, and Elmer turned to me and said, "They're pretty funny, ain't they?"

"I been listenin' to them for so many years now," I replied. "They always make me laugh."

It was a fairly uneventful drive, and we made pretty good time, reaching the Minnesota border about midafternoon. We'd had our lunch some time back and were now stopped for a leg stretch and a look around at one of Elmer's "fishin' holes"—a large, somewhat decrepit building at the edge of a small border town that was a stationary, year-round flea market. I remember Elmer guiding me into a stop, saying it was a good place.

"What they got in there?" I asked him.

"Got everything in there," he said, getting out of the cab.

We went in, and he wasn't lying. It was one of those places that wasn't a pawn shop, but in rural America serves much the same function. People with something to sell bring it in, and if the owner likes it, he buys it and resells it. Everything from old pots and pans, tools, linens, traps, and appliances to movies, books, and buckets. I remember he bought a bunch of matching ashtrays for the ceremony house that was to be built, and I got an old factory-made blanket, red and gray, with a generic "Indian" design on it and a copy of Peter S. Beagle's *I See by My Outfit*, a favorite of mine.

We got to the Pipestone National Monument by late afternoon, just before they closed. There was the usual info desk, events kiosk, and shelves and shelves of Indian-made things in the gift shop, including more beautiful *canunpas* than I've ever seen anywhere. In the rear display areas, past the historical presentation section, there was only one Native pipe carver at work. He was a Dakota-lookin' guy who took one look at me, with my blond hair, and turned surly. He wouldn't speak or even acknowledge our presence. Luckily, one of the park rangers brought us an armload of stone, so we didn't have to deal with Mr. Surly.

Elmer was grinning as we left, obviously pleased to have been so well treated, and as we headed out, we saw posted flyers advertising a powwow close by. We stopped at a small highway diner for supper, and the most memorable thing about it was that there was obviously a Renaissance Fair going on somewhere in the area. Various outlaws, knights, ladies, and oafs were seated around us, and as we began with our coffee, one young transvestite came in, complete with powder and wig, stomacher and farthingale, and a hoop-rigged gown, the whole giving the effect of a tall-masted ship under full sail. Dinner and a show!

We checked into a Super 8 before we hit the powwow, and after we'd checked in and were nearly to our room, I found a two-dollar bill blown against the next room's door. Elmer had just been saying we'd gotten a good deal on our room. Since I spotted the bill first, I claimed it by scooping it up. He stopped, squinted at me, and exclaimed, "You lucky."

The sun was setting when we left the motel, and it was approaching twilight when we got to the powwow. There was just enough light left for us to make our rounds of the vendors' stalls. I don't recall which tribe was sponsoring the event, or who all the drum groups were, but it was a good-sized dance arena. I remember Elmer wanted to buy a nice set of several drumsticks for use in monthly ceremony but was hesitant until I offered to help out.

"You want cheep in?" he asked.

"Sure," I responded.

So he got what he wanted "for the people," and I bought several types of beads, some hair pipes, some repro red chevrons, some small brass ones, an abalone disc, and some artificial sinew. I also found some hand-carved bone eagle feathers, about the right size for a pair of earrings, and a small carved-stone frog. I dithered a bit over a buffalo skull, which I would have painted and donated to the sun dance, but they wanted too much for it— and it wasn't even a bull's. "Them bull skulls, they got a bump, like, in middle of here," Elmer said, indicating the center of the forehead with his finger. "This one's cow."

So, laden with our purchases, we refreshed ourselves with hot coffee and fry bread and went to the grandstands to watch the dancers. We were just in time for the grand entry now that it was dark, and the management had turned on the big lights. I remember the young ladies' butterfly dances were extremely graceful, and the dancers in the Men's Traditional category were exceptionally well decked out in authentic-looking regalia. The drums were good, always keeping an even, fast beat, and although I can't recall any of the arena director's patter, he called the drums and dances well.

Elmer told me he used to dance competitively in the Men's Traditional until one time, a rival for first place had been so angered by Elmer beating him, he'd blown with his breath a little bad-medicine dart into Elmer's right knee, and Elmer had never been a first-class dancer since. I mentioned this incident earlier on, but this was the occasion of Elmer's telling me about it himself.

As the judges strode back to the announcer's stand, after having closely watched the dancers, Elmer indicated one young man out near the front. "I think that one, he's gonna get that first money." I'd been watching the same dancer, and though I was— and remain—ignorant of the finer points, I agreed. And indeed, that dancer took first place.

That night in the motel room, we just relaxed. Elmer lay back on his bed, smoking and not saying much. We had cable TV, and there was a *Star Trek* marathon on the Sci-Fi Channel. I was busy with my beads. The pattern of brass, chevrons, spacers, and hair pipes was shaping up into a nice choker, and I kept at it 'til lights-out. I was able to finish it that night, except for the center disc. I had to Krazy Glue the frog and the two bone feathers on later.

The next morning, we had a quick coffee and snack in the lobby and hit the road home. I recall we stopped midmorning at a little roadside café to which Elmer had directed me. It was a little off the main highway, and as we went in, it was just like the old Firesign Theatre line: "We looked around, and there was nothing but Indians!" We ordered some more coffee and a bite to eat and sat down. There were contemporary Native sounds on the system, and I really dug the place, but not a soul would look at me or even acknowledge my existence. This was an Indian joint, and probably being there with Elmer was the only reason I was tolerated at all. It's hard to begrudge the people wanting to have something all their own. I've read Native authors bewailing the fact that there's no place or circumstances where the *wasicus* won't intrude their unwanted selves. It's hard not to sympathize, even though it means cutting myself out, at least potentially, from a scene where I've found so much power and meaning.

We were soon on the road again, and the only other notable stop was midafternoon, when I found myself zoning out behind the wheel and had to pull over to a wayside rest area to spread out my blanket by the truck and get in a catnap. Then it was back to Rosebud and Elmer's double-wide.

A little later on in the year, I again drove Elmer to Minnesota, but this time to do ceremony in a church basement. His trailer was still parked at his old place in Ironwood, and the family squatters there had been giving him a hard time. I recall that once, during a sweat before monthly ceremony, Irene's young son had been down in the woods along the bottom, firing off his .22 rifle just to harass us. A young white woman had been staying with Elmer after Maidcha returned to Germany, and she was trying to protect him, but it was too much for her. That later trip to the Twin Cities was uneventful, and recalling it reminds me I was up in Rosebud quite a few times that winter of 2000/01.

Later on in the winter, perhaps in late January, an Indian man whose name escapes me was there with Elmer when I arrived with a load of groceries. Once again, the ladies at Warehouse Surplus in Wahoo had gifted me with extra items, once they knew I was going up to the rez to help out. I recall it was a gray winter afternoon when I pulled in, and this man and Elmer were sitting in the trailer's kitchen, smoking and having coffee. I may be confusing separate visits, but this was the weekend when the power went out. It wasn't a ceremony weekend; I'd come up a week early to hang out and spend some time making myself useful, and now here was someone before me. Well, we had a good time 'til that evening, when a storm took out a major power line. Luckily, the trailer was hooked up to gas for heat, and I was able to scrounge a candle out of my truck, but it got pretty dark that weekend. Elmer seemed unconcerned and remarked that this happened pretty often in winter.

It wasn't until late the next morning, Sunday, when the lights came back on and we were able to watch TV again. I must have made three or four visits that winter, and I think my memories here are a fusing of the first two.

At about this time, some of the older and senior sun dancers had donated materials, time, and labor and had begun construction on a new ceremony house that would also serve as a cook-shack. Winter had halted its construction; it lay there half-built. But I remember I went away with a mission: to get a woodstove for it once it was done.

Early that spring, so early it was still snowy, there was another trip to Minneapolis. The Indian man I'd just met and the white woman who still came around to help Elmer, although she was no longer full-time, accompanied us up there to see Grandma Darlene and have dinner in a Vietnamese restaurant before the ceremony. I happened to travel to the restaurant in another car with Grandma Dar. When Elmer, the white girl, and the Indian guy arrived, she was spittin' mad. She said the man had left Elmer unattended for a little while, on a public street, while he went off to do something that was entirely his own affair. He was pretty sheepish about it, and it was the beginning of the end for him. After that trip, he didn't come around Elmer's anymore.

I also remember that I had a ceremonial pipe I was planning to use in sun dance, and it was brought out for use in this ceremony. On one return trip from a powwow during my marriage, I had stopped off for a road break at a highway mall that contained an antique mall. I went in, and instead of looking around the main gallery, I made a sharp left from the front door and found myself in the booth of a vendor who obviously specialized in Native artifacts. In the case directly before me was a stone effigy pipe, a frog, carved from Cherokee greenstone. I bought it and made a bag for it of white buckskin, and my ex donated a stem that fit it perfectly. After our split, I made another stem and tried and tried to carve the end to fit the tapered socket, but I could never get it right. We used that pipe in ceremony that night. The young lady was the pipe holder, but she told me later the pipe had come loose during the ceremony.

The light was very dim in the church basement where ceremony was held, even prior to its being extinguished completely during ceremony. I remember that girl stood with her legs straight, head held high, almost in a defiant pose, tryin' to get it right. Then the frog fell off. We put it back on and continued the ceremony, but the nose had suffered some slight damage on hitting the tile floor, and although I may have prayed with it once or twice since, and decorated the bag with some fantastic heavy greenstone beads, I have since discontinued using it. I'd tried and tried to carve the stem to fit the peculiar, sloping inverted cone that was the socket, but no luck. Even wrapping the stem's end with sinew hadn't helped.

I made at least two more trips up to visit Elmer before spring that year. One was a trip during the coldest, snowiest part of winter. I'd found an old, fairly heavy, medium-sized wood-burning stove that was chambered and piped for a water heater. I thought it would make a good stove for the new ceremony house. I only recall some discrete incidents from this trip. One was a moment early on after my arrival. This may have been for the January or February ceremony. Elmer had received a bizarre, almost demented letter from some guy who had been known to him at some prior time. The text was rambling, incoherent, and alluded to the writer wondering if he should commit fatal violence against a woman he knew; the whole thing was palpably the product of someone who'd lost his grip. It angered Elmer to have been sent such a thing. He showed it to me, let me read it, and sat down in his chair in disgust. I scanned it, looked up, and said, "Elmer, you don't have to answer this. It's too crazy. Just throw it away, or burn it."

He didn't say anything right away but looked relieved. It had really peeved him. "Why he send me this?"

This visit and the siting and interrupted construction of the new ceremony house took place at Elmer's new homesite. His double-wide had been purchased used for him by the tribe, but it still had a few moves left in it, despite its early 1970s vintage. He was now at a remove of two or three miles from the Ironwood homesite, his son Norman's outfit. He had gone there to get away from Irene and her bunch of squatters in his old house and didn't yet have the TV aerial set up. The weekend I was there,

there was a young Lakota fellow hangin' out, and we'd gone into Mission and bought a new aerial and cable. There was a hole to be dug and a post to be set for the antenna mast. I think I got in Thursday evening, and we went to Mission on Friday, but we somehow spaced off getting this work done until Saturday evening. There was snow on the ground and it was already dark outside when we heard a knock on the door. Another young Lakota man stepped aside, shut the door, and turned and said, "Hello." Everyone started laughing, since he'd accented his pronunciation of the word to sound like someone who knew what to say, but not being an English speaker, said it with a strong Indian accent and made it sound like he knew this was the correct noise to make but didn't really know the word. It's a hard kind of joke to describe, but even though I'd never heard anyone else do this before, I got it and knew why everyone else was laughing.

Well, we sat around on the living room floor that evening, with Elmer in his easy chair, smoking his nearly ever-present Camels, with his definitely ever-present wide-bottomed coffee mug, obviously enjoying all the company. We were studying the instructions for the new TV aerial, which left me boggled. I turned it over to one of the other young men. Not much went on during that visit, but it was good to have sober company on a cold winter's night.

To backtrack once again, there had been a time, earlier in the autumn, when Johnson, one of Elmer's sons, had shown up drunk at his dad's with a couple of his drunk buddies. They all trooped in, Johnson bold as brass and the other guys looking scared, and sat down, whereupon Johnson had declared his intention to spend some time with his dad, singing old-time songs. Elmer wouldn't stand for it. "You guys goin' 'round every day gettin' drunk, hah? Ever fuckin' day!" That was the only time I'd ever heard the old man drop the f-bomb and the first time I ever saw him so angry.

The others didn't wait. They took off outside, jumped in their pickup, and left Johnson stuck without a ride. By now, it was obvious his first plan wasn't going to fly, so he asked me to give him a ride to an address in a little rez town some miles away, where his girlfriend lived. I didn't like leaving the old man alone, but it was worth it to get Johnson out of there before he brought the spirits' wrath down on his father. When we arrived at his girlfriend's, he actually tried to get me to get out of my pickup and go see if she was in. Not only was this a bad idea, a strange white man knocking on someone's door after dark, but it definitely didn't fit in with my plan of ditching him there. I refused, saying, "No, look, Johnson, she doesn't know me, and besides she's your girlfriend, not mine."

He obviously expected to be dumped, for he left the passenger door open a crack as he got out. I wasted no time—turned the engine on, shut and locked doors, and reversed out of there. I don't think he'd even made it to the front door by the time I was tooling out the drive. It reminded me of the time in Santee when Patti had said to Jamie, "Why don't you live on the rez, instead of payin' rent to some *wasicu*?" or some such.

He'd replied, "'Cause I don't want to spend my time runnin' off drunks."

I regret to say that the alcoholic, substance-influenced, dysfunctional reservation culture that had grown up in Indian country—and almost totally supplanted the traditional ways of the people—must now become an ever-present backdrop, and occasional key element, in the rest of the stories I have about my time with Elmer.

Winter Journeys

THIS GET-TOGETHER MUST HAVE TAKEN PLACE SOON AFTER the items' recovery but before the second of the winter's visits. I remember two little scenes from each: One is Elmer just sitting in his chair, smoking and looking out the window at the vast sweep of prairie, now blanketed in snow to the far line of pines along the banks of a stream, miles away. Everything was utterly still in the way only possible far from the city and without power. Not even the sound of a passing vehicle on the highway reached us. For a moment, it was like stepping back in time a century or so.

The second is from the visit with all the company. I had run into Mission once again, after the weekend, to buy a simple recording system from Radio Shack—an amp, cassette deck, microphone, and speakers so Elmer could record some of his songs. I recall that by this time, only one of the visitors was left, a Lakota man younger than I was, and together we got the system set up and got Elmer to start recording. Then I had to leave the next morning.

After the trips to the Twin Cities and the winter visits, my next visit was the rainy, cold, and muddy time of the year that was no longer winter but not yet spring. I may have missed monthly ceremony in February, but I recall that the weather was still quite cool, cold at nights. I'd been spending some time with my pup and the new kitten I'd gotten in January from my Nebraska neighbor Jim. He was retired and lived next door with his wife, so it was no trouble for him to feed and spend some time with them when I was gone.

I'd been in a bit of a hurry to get away, and while my monthly prayer ties and altar ties were done and hanging on the west wall of the small front room where I kept my ceremonial things, I'd neglected to make my travel ties. Just two short strings of six red ones each, to be hung fore and aft in whatever vehicle, but I left without them. I figured, hey, I'm up to see the *wicasa wakan*, with a load of groceries and tobacco—what could happen? Well, I found out. Without specific protection from the spirits, I was vulnerable. Just as I crossed the Mission city limits, an oncoming truck's tire threw a chunk of gravel right in line with my face. Bam! It starred the windshield but good. Since then, I've never driven any distance without travel ties.

However, I cannot seem to recall much from that visit. I made the long trip from Nebraska to Rosebud so many times that year. The reminiscences of the winter's visits sort of blur together, and those of the spring seem even vaguer. I recall how damp it was the whole time, how the toilet paper in the outhouse absorbed the moisture in the air and turned soggy and disintegrated in your hand as you were trying to use it.

Now another memory of the previous autumn comes to mind. It was after that young woman who had tried to stay by Elmer when he was on his own old property at Ironwood had finally been run off by his relatives.

The oldest of Irene's boys, the one with the .22 rifle, had finally managed to terrorize her into leaving, and he had Elmer scared. One evening, before the trip for the doctoring ceremony in Minneapolis, we heard shots from close by. Apparently, whenever Elmer had a visitor who might come between him and his family's victimizations, they tried to scare them in this way. I didn't mind it too much, but it rattled the old man. He had a set of arrows and a bow, a light sports model, that he was keeping with him in his bedroom. A security light had been installed near his double-wide, but they'd shot it out, so things were pretty dark. I wasn't yet asleep on the living-room couch when Elmer came up out of his bedroom, which was nearest the old house, and brought some bedding and the bow with him. I took the floor and gave him the couch when he explained he was going to sleep at this end of the trailer, for fear of being shot. What with the alcohol and the drugging going on next door, it was quite understandable.

This next trip was still later in the spring. After a long day's drive, we were just in view of the Twin Cities when a terrific thunderstorm burst overhead. It was a Friday evening. For those of you who don't know, traffic in and around the Twin Cities on any evening is bad, but on a Friday evening, it's a nightmare. People seem to just go crazy and lose any regard for other drivers. I remember having a real hard time following Elmer's directions while fighting the traffic as the thunder and lightning cracked right overhead. *This is it,* I thought. *I've had it with this shit. This is absolutely the last time.* And so on.

Well, Elmer directed me to a private home where we were fed and each given a bunk; mine was the couch. It was a Native family whose father was one of Elmer's dancers. Not too shabby, except I was having trouble getting my head on straight after freaking out in the traffic and the storm. I'd lost a hearing aid on the way in from the pickup, which made conversation difficult—and, to top it off, with the weather being so bad, there weren't enough people stirring. So Elmer said to me, sitting at these folks' kitchen table with his cigarette and cup of coffee, "No ceremony at this time."

However, the trip was far from being a waste, for we looked up Grandma Darlene, and she got us into the AIM Sun Dance at Pipestone. At least, I recall being there with her, being the only white guy there, and feeling pretty gratified at finding myself in the same room with John Trudell. He was with a group of Basque separatists, the ETA group. So this trip must have been later on in the summer.

Earlier in the year, I was again back up in Rosebud, at Elmer's new location at Norman and Shannon's for monthly ceremony. I recall that we had gone over to Gilli's to have him sign a document relating to some family business. Gilli was at his girlfriend's house, a little BIA prefab. At first, he was reluctant to sign and tried to put his dad off, saying he'd sign it later.

But Elmer wasn't having it. "I'm the only dad you got," he admonished him.

Finally, the Lakota lady got up and made a sort of a high-pitched growl at Gilli, obviously wishing him to sign and get it done. Well, he finally did, and we left.

Our next stop was at the tribal fire station in Rosebud, the original reservation settlement. Elmer needed some land-use documents signed—to do with harvesting sage and pine boughs on open tribal land for the sun dance. We had to wait for most of the lunch hour, 'til the fire marshal got back. Finally, it was on up to the legal aid office in Mission so Elmer could file his papers and talk to a lawyer about cutting all ties with Patti. This took another good while, but when he came out, he was obviously relieved. He said it was all taken care of, then dropped a bombshell on me. I'd been to the county courthouse in Winner before, sometime, so I knew the location he meant when he told me that when he and Patti had gotten together, she had at one point insisted on his marrying her for reasons best known to herself. She'd gone into the courthouse by herself while he'd stayed out in the pickup quite a while. "When she came out, she said, 'Okay we're married,'" Elmer said. "But I don't think that's right, 'cause I never did it."

I was dumbstruck at first. "Elmer, that's right. If you didn't say it in front of a justice of the peace, or a judge, you didn't do it. You're not married."

I couldn't believe it. All those years she'd been with him in Santee, calling herself "Mrs. Running," and the rest of it—how she'd told me the elders had approved of her being with Elmer, going out of her way to impress me and others that she was the medicine man's especial confidante, and, not incidentally, sharing in the prestige and spoils, such as they were. At least she'd kept the drunks away; I have to give her that. And she prevented certain people from picking the old man over like a vulture tearing into a fresh roadkill. Since I've already told how negligent and abusive she became just before he returned to Rosebud, I won't go over that again.

My next trip up must have been for the monthly ceremony in May. I recall getting there a few days early so I'd have some time to spend with him. The recording equipment I'd bought had disappeared, unfortunately, and with all I saw happen since, I'm afraid it must have been stolen to pay for one or the other of his boys' drunks. I recall him telling me that some of the other sun dancers had been up there to visit and help out. They'd had a good time until just about suppertime, when one of the younger kids from Irene's came over to tell him in Lakota that there was nothing to eat over to home. Elmer replied briefly in Lakota, and the kid took off. After telling me the story, Elmer turned to me and said, "You take alla them cans, bread, coffee, everything in that closet"—pointing to the large kitchen cupboard—"and some meat in that Frigidaire. Take it all over to Irene's."

Now, the big multishelved pantry was absolutely chock-full. As I said, other sun dancers had been by and left their contributions: crackers, coffee, sugar, oil, bread, some canned vegetables, pickles, mustard, ketchup, and other condiments galore—the usual contents, but almost overflowing. Burger and bacon in the freezer. I did what I was told, got some boxes, filled 'em up, put 'em in the back of my pickup, and drove the few hundred yards over to Irene's. When I knocked at the back door, a voice from within bade me enter. I had with me the box with the burger and bread on top.

Irene was sitting in the kitchen with one of her friends or relations, smoking. She asked me, "What's this?" kind of suspiciously.

I told her Elmer was sending the food over. When I said this and set the box down on the table and they looked inside, the young boy who'd come over got a wildly happy expression and started hugging me around the knees and dancing.

Irene and her company lost their attitudes in a big way, and it was all smiles and *wopilas*.

I said, "You're welcome," and went out to get the rest of the stuff.

By the time I'd brought in the last load, Irene was at the range, frying up some burger that hadn't been frozen.

They all said their thank-yous in Lakota again, and that kitchen was full of some very expectant-looking children.

I got back to Elmer's trailer, and he was sitting at the kitchen table where I'd left him, just smoking, with his coffee cup at his elbow, not saying a word. I likewise kept silent. That was one of the things about Grandpa: He taught mostly by example, the old way, and said more in his silence than most folks can jabbering their heads off. I knew he'd been terrorized by Irene and her bunch, that they'd been making his life more difficult than it already was—and for a traditional medicine man, it's plenty hard enough to start off with. Nonetheless, he was keeping the ways of his people. When it came to hungry kids, he minded the hostility no more than he would a dog lifting his leg against his lodgepole.

I know all comparisons are invidious, but I have to say I've met some folks—who weren't shy of letting me know how Christian they were—who would have felt perfectly justified in letting those who'd wronged them go without.

Well, all that was left in the house was what I'd brought. I can't recall what we had for supper ourselves, but the next morning I made us bacon and eggs with toast. Afterward, when I announced that I was finding my knife a trifle dull, Elmer put a little whetstone on the countertop. I'd always kept a nice Buck or Schrade Old Timer with me whenever I was working with Grandpa on the rez since it came in handy so often. "There," he said. "You could use that, whenever you want, sharp' you knife."

I said, *"Pilamaye."*

And he went on, apropos of my also having mentioned getting a shower: "Good thing you chase away you porcupine buddy. I want you to drive me over to medicine-man meetin' at that casino."

So off we went. When we entered the big casino building just over the Nebraska–South Dakota line, I was stopped by security, who told me I couldn't wear my knife in its belt sheath into the casino. As we passed through the plush and sumptuous lobby, I called Elmer's attention to a beautiful, fire-engine-red Indian Chief motorcycle parked there. It was being raffled off as a casino promo. Apparently, it was the same model used by the star of a TV series about an Indian detective who rode around solving crimes.

Elmer said, "I got a couple tickets on that."

"If you win it," I told him, "I'll trade you my new Chevy pickup for it, straight across."

"OK, bring it over. Just fill up the tank with gas."

When we got into the big reserved room off the main floor, there were several long tables set up with chairs and a large buffet being made ready. Carafes of water stood at each table, and there was the smell of coffee brewing. The meeting began shortly after we arrived and sat down. The main concerns being aired were the harvesting of sage and pine boughs for the various sun dances. Also, the presence of non-Native sun dancers. The increasing scarcity of sage was discussed, with the chairman calling one speaker's attention to the fact that in the 1940s and 1950s, "This reservation was covered with sage." The correct method of picking it came up, which is to cut the stem and leave the root, and not to pick after the (remaining) plants had gone to seed. There was also some discussion about growing it. At least one person called attention to the fact that money wasn't supposed to be charged for it. The plant was there free to benefit the people, and the real reason for its growing scarcity was just that.

One disturbing thing was an account given by one of the few women present, an elder who told us how a pickup load of young men, some non-Native, had come onto a remote part of her allotment without permission and been videotaped illegally cutting pine boughs. When she'd challenged them, they'd shouted out that it was for a sun dance. They disregarded her verbal notice that they were trespassing and had even shouted abuse and given her the finger as they left. Some of this footage was shown on a big TV monitor. This led to a discussion of traditional values being lost, such as respect for the elderly, and then to the subject of non-Native participation in the sun dance.

Elmer had kept quiet until now, but at this point he spoke up. "Most of you here know me. I been runnin' sun dance for more than twenty years. We use quite a bit of sage for that. When the spirits told me to put up a sun-dance grounds for the people, they didn't say, 'Just for the Indian people.' I keep my white sun dancers along with me all the time. There's one of 'em sittin' right there," he said, pointing at me.

He went on to say a bit more about how the sage was put on the Mother Earth so the people could have good health and help, and about how, when the pine boughs came off his arbor, he sent them down to Crow Dog's so they could be used again. I kind of lost track of his exact flow, though, after he focused the room's attention on me. It's hard to describe, being the only white man in a big roomful of not just Indians but of medicine men and *ikce wicasa*.

I kept my head down and my eyes on the table in front of me, trying to be humble and respectful. I knew that any one of these men was the intimate of powers that, if he chose to, he could make almost anything happen. The moderator began his closing remarks after Elmer spoke his piece. Again, the intensity of self-consciousness kinda wiped out my memory of them. Then the meeting was done, the buffet was ready, and I and one other young(er) person were asked to serve the eldest present, which we did.

I recall one elderly gentleman in particular; he nodded gently in approval as I set his plate down in front of him. His striking feature was his nose. It was the most unique specimen I've ever encountered. Broad at the base, it swelled majestically to a sharp Roman declivity, whence it tapered to a sharp point. On the whole, it bore a disturbing resemblance to a sweet potato.

The lunch was pretty good, and the meeting broke up soon after. Elmer and I headed back, and that evening, he and I did one of the few fun things together of our association. Not that being around him and working with him wasn't fun—it was. I mean, a thing done for fun on its own. We went to the county fair.

This must have been after the monthly ceremony in May, for I remember the sweetness of the evening air, the fact that it was still getting dark early, and the beginning of the summer's dryness. After the snowmelt and the spring rains, there's not much precipitation in South Dakota until October.

We got there just after sundown, but neither of us was much interested in the rides, so we just sauntered along the midway, checking out the amusements. Elmer had shaved before we left and was dressed in his best black jeans, black cowboy shirt and boots, and fringed black leather vest. He was enjoying himself, even though we weren't really taking part in the fair. We stopped and talked to two young men, carnies who were doing some mechanical work on one of the rides that lay idle. I don't recall much of what was said, but Elmer and the two, well, *boys*, they seemed to me, were having a swell time just shooting the breeze, telling him which rides had broken down recently, which had caused an injury to a fairgoer, where they'd been playing, how long they'd been with the show, and so on.

I seem to recall Elmer introducing himself as a medicine man, which he would do sometimes. He was enjoying their willingness to share their stories with him. He could, and did, spend some days alone in the trailer without complaining, but he was a pretty sociable person. He really enjoyed people.

That was a weeknight around monthly ceremony in May, I believe. One of the things I've left out, which was such a constant feature of life with the old medicine man, was the ritual of the spirit plate. At every mealtime, except when we were on the road, a little bit of the foodstuffs being served would be put in a little dish or small plate, before eating. It got to be a regular saying at those times: "I've fed the spirits, so it's OK." At intervals of no more than four days, usually more often, the plate would be taken outside and offered to Wakan Tanka, to those above, to the four winds, and to the Mother Earth and those below. The idea was the same as that behind all such offerings, to show thanks for the food, and to feed any hungry spirits that might be around. Even such a small thing as this can be the first step to getting the spirits' attention. Those interested should see the movie *Thunderheart*.

I made breakfast again that morning, the new moon, and by the time it came to sweat, there were quite a few people there. A couple of lady sun-dance leaders were there to run sweat for the women who came, and Elmer ran it for the guys. I remember that was a hard one. I managed to make it through all four doors, but just barely. After everyone had crawled outside and shaken hands, several of us just crawled around to the back of the lodge and laid out on our towels, waiting for the sky to stop whirling around. I noticed Elmer, now in his early eighties, just walked over to his pickup, opened the door, changed back into his jeans and work shirt, tucked his eagle-wing fan onto the dash, picked up his travel mug and took a sip, and lit a cigarette as if nothing were any different.

Well, hell, I remember thinking groggily. *If I had a bunch of powerful spirits helping me, maybe I wouldn't be lying here, either.* Then I sat up and lit a smoke of my own. There's nothing like that first smoke after sweat.

Ceremony went late that night. I seem to remember there were several doctorings, and we didn't get to the feasting 'til 3:00 a.m. I was tucked away in a far corner of the living room, and Elmer was looking for me after the lights went back on. There was some laughter when I called out to let him know I was there. "Oh, you made it! You was over there!" he exclaimed.

I had gotten into the habit of skipping out on ceremony after running the fire and sweating sometimes, just because I was tired and didn't want to stay up half the night. But not this time.

CHAPTER 12

A Bitter Spring

THE NEXT TRIP TO ELMER'S WASN'T SO GOOD. I'D FOUND A
stylish black jean jacket with laced-up slits in the sides,
showy vents, and silver grommets and buttons. It was cut very
swag. I'd only had it a few days before I arrived for a sun-dance
meeting in early June. As soon as I walked in the door, Elmer was
all over it. He wanted to trade for it. It was the first time I had a
mind to tell the old man no—and I still wish I had. I've regretted
letting it go ever since. He had a few jackets that were big enough
for me, and I traded away the new one. But I didn't really care for
the one I picked and gave it away as soon as I got home.

Gilli was there, and he left before the meeting. He borrowed
Elmer's pickup and was supposed to return it by the weekend.
A lot of the sun-dance leaders showed up, men and women, as
well as some of the longtimers, folks I remembered from Santee.
We had a good meeting. Elmer chastised us at first, more out of
form, I think, than anything else. "Look at you. Drinkin' coffee,
smokin' cigarettes!" It was a case of look who's talking, but no
one said so. There was affection for him; you could feel it in the
room. He concluded his remarks by saying the sun dancers were
"all my kids." The meeting itself was boring, and the only thing
I remember was afterward, when one of the longtimers called

me on a little blue Buddhist figurine I was wearing around my neck. It was actually a feminine sky goddess, Dakini, but I didn't correct him when he asked me why I was "wearing a Buddha." I responded that I was wearing it simply because I liked it, but I've always wished that I'd said, "Saints presarve us. They're always after me lucky charrums!"

Well, they all left after a day of cleaning up the sweat lodges and clearing brush around the sun-dance arbor. There was no sweat at that time, but someone had brought in a load of wood and even one of rocks. I remember being there alone with the old man on Monday morning after the weekend meeting was done. Gilli came in afoot, without the pickup truck, and as hung over as a road-killed skunk. He just barged right in, muttered something to his dad, and right in front of us proceeded to open the drawers in the living-room bureau, rummage around, pull something out, and leave. I recall Elmer looked scared. I got a little hot, but figured the best thing was to let him go.

We had to go get Elmer's truck out of the rez impound. Apparently, Gilli had been picked up for drunk driving and then spent the weekend in the tank. A few of the sun dancers who were staying in town showed up later on to do a little more work on the arbor. I left just after they arrived, since the old man wasn't all alone. I was mad about the jacket, fed up with Elmer's tolerance of Gilli's victimizing him, and disgusted with the fact that I'd had to cover the fine at impound lot. I left pretty early, just after the men went up to work, and I had to pay for my abruptness at the next monthly ceremony.

I got there a couple of days early, and there were some of the other sun dancers there. One of the first things Elmer asked me was, "You gonna stay around?"

I told him I would, and later on, one of those who'd been there when I'd taken off before said, "We didn't know you'd left. Somebody said you weren't around, and Elmer said, 'He's proba-

bly up at the sun-dance grounds, workin',' but then we saw your
vehicle was gone."

I tried to explain about how I was starting to get burned out,
mostly talking about how Gilli had been behaving and treating
the old man badly, without saying much about the jacket trade.

If I remember right, this seemed to be accepted at face value,
and since I'd brought in a load of groceries and a carton of smokes
for the old man, as I usually did, no more was said.

The sweat that time wasn't as hard as the one before. I recall
lots of people were there. After we'd finished covering up the big
hall mirror and the windows in the trailer, and saged the food,
and Elmer had his altar set up, I was a short ways down the hall,
off the living room, lined up and sitting next to a young Lakota
mother and her small child. I remember I was a little tired and
cranky, but when a fellow came down the hall distributing sprigs
of sage for everyone to wear behind their left ear, I picked up the
one I honestly thought was meant for me—and since it was one of
the big ones I'd brought from the large patch outside Valentine, I
broke it in two, just as the young lady said, "That's mine."

Well, that got things off to an awkward start. I offered her
the pieces, but she waved me off. Then her child (I couldn't tell if
it was a boy or a girl) began staring fixedly at me until I'd raise
my eyes and look back. It was weird, and it made things worse.
This went on, look and away, back and forth, three or four times,
until the mother got disgusted, picked up her kid, and quietly
stormed out. I felt like shit about it. From zero to fuckup in under
three minutes. I was probably the only one there who knew she
was storming, she was so tight-lipped about it, but I felt like the
typical, ignorant *wasicu* bastard who doesn't know enough of the
old ways to be able to respect them but still wants to be there—a
persona against which I had sedulously striven to personify. No,
I'd never wanted to personify that persona or be that guy, but

there it was done, at least to that mother and child, and I don't really recall much more of that ceremony or the visit.

I recall there was one incident, sometime before the sun-dance meeting, when Elmer's family friction came to a head. This was before the move to Norman's. Someone had either called the tribal police about the kid of Irene's with the .22 rifle—who had actually run off one or two of the sun dancers who were volunteering their labor on the sun-dance grounds at Ironwood—or Irene may have gotten wind of Elmer's going to legal aid, trying to clarify title to the land. I remember we discussed ways and means of getting her and the rest out of Elmer's old house. Anyway, she came storming over one afternoon, mad as a wet hen, and demanded to use the phone, since she didn't have one and this was just before cheap TracFones and minute cards became available on the rez.

She called up one of her relatives in White River, a reservation some miles to the north, and told someone there to tell so-and-so to get his rifle and come on down. "Gonna shoot me some Runnings!" she spat into the receiver and stormed out again. Unbelievable, using the phone of the party you were on the warpath against. I kinda think this happened before the time Elmer told me to take the groceries over to feed her and her kids. Things smoothed out after that, at least on the surface, and I recall sometime around my visit in June, she actually came over for a neighborly visit with Elmer. I'd brought a Weedwacker and some other implements for the sweat and for grounds keeping, because, as I mentioned during my stay in Santee, Grandpa was very particular about his sun-dance grounds and keeping the sweat lodge areas neat. No weeds or tall grass allowed, and there was always a coffee can for cigarette butts at each of the benches between the lodges. Anyhow, there Elmer and Irene sat, smoking and chatting in Lakota, while I took the Weedwacker around to the back of the trailer so as not to disturb them with its noise. I can still see them sitting in the late afternoon South Dakota sunshine—two old Lakota people, sitting in straight-backed chairs, both of them looking off into different aspects of the distance, exchanging remarks.

Once again I feel I have to revise my time line; it must have been around the June monthly ceremony that the above took place, and July when the incident with the sprig of sage took place, since sage doesn't start to get tall until later on in July. I remember just before the July monthly ceremony, several of the older sun dancers had brought in bundles of sage, but none of it was as tall as the bunch I'd found. It was simply too early for the sage to have been that tall in June. These stalks were twelve to fourteen inches long, whilst theirs were only ten or so. One of the senior dancers remarked on it, and it was my picking up and breaking one of these longer ones that sparked the incident. So, the (temporary) reconciliation with Irene must have been a little earlier.

I remember taking a road trip up north with the old man, past White River sometime that spring, and several trips into Valentine. We were on a hardware-store run there once and ran into the venerable Rosebud Grandma, who was the holder of Grandpa's pipe for ceremony and sun dance that year. I can't recall her name, though we'd all been introduced to her during the sun-dance meeting. There she was in the old Coast to Coast Hardware. She didn't speak any English—at least, I never heard her do so. In the Lakota way, as I understand it, a woman of respectable standing is needed to hold the *canunpa* for the medicine man and so stand in for the White Buffalo Calf Woman, who brought the sacred pipe to the people. If I'm getting any of this wrong, my humble apologies. The fault is mine. But as with his conversation with Irene, I can see the two of them, pleasantly surprised at the chance meeting, smiling in the busy shop, her in her shawl and long dress, Elmer in his black vest, jeans, cowboy boots, and cap, talking Indian to each other, as the old man would say. He really took pains with his appearance whenever we went to town; he'd shave, change clothes, and clean out his glass eye.

Not to toot my own horn, but there were occasions when Elmer commended me to some of the sun dancers and his family. To Norman, I believe it was, he said, "Karl's a good driver," when the subject of the road trips came up. And again, "Karl's a good cook," to some of the dancers at the meeting. Since cooking is traditionally the woman's job, in the old ways, this was almost an occasion for a few joking remarks directed at me. (Just like when Elmer's spirits may have told him that some of the men weren't gonna make it all the way through sweat: "Patti!" he'd call. "Get some you dresses for these guys; they ain't gon' make it all the way.") Almost, but not quite; I was spared the teasing on that occasion at least.

But some teasing came up once in a way I didn't much like. Upon hearing that I was the beneficiary of a trust fund and had no need of a work routine, when the subject of my frequent visits came up, one of the old-timers said, "I can't even imagine what that's like."

Another one said, "Man, if I didn't have to work, I'd spend all my time up here with the medicine man, taking care of him."

I wish he'd known better than to say that. Not only is life on the rez no picnic for anybody, as far as I can see, but that's a type of decision that's almost in the marriage category—deciding how and with whom you're going to spend the foreseeable future. No one has the right to attempt to sway another's decision on such a serious thing. I can see the appeal, though, to thinking that: Moving there to take care of Elmer would have taken the strain of obligation off a lot of people. Anyway, I didn't have anything to say to that remark. I believe that one-sided exchange took place around July ceremony time, which brings me up to August and sun dance of 2001.

Well, I got there a day or two before purification, with the usual groceries and smokes for the old man, my prayer ties and flags, and other paraphernalia for going up on the hill and dancing, and stuff for giveaway for my fourth-year *wopila*, or thanking. I found out that, ordinarily, one is supposed to do four days lamenting, as the *hanblechiya* is properly translated, every year before one sun dances, and I'd never even been up once! And this was to be my fourth year! So I parked my vehicle and set up camp in one of the very few places at Ironwood where there was at least a prospect of shade, even if only in the early mornings. It was just to the west of the little slope that led down to the cook-shack. I asked Elmer if that was OK, and he said yeah.

CHAPTER 13

The Wrong Reasons

UNFORTUNATELY, THE PURIFICATION AND SUN DANCE WERE beset from the beginning by the friction and struggle for control between Elmer and Irene. The first day of getting my camp set up, here comes a Lakota woman, someone I'd never seen before, telling me I couldn't camp there because it was the favored spot of another family. When I responded that Elmer had told me it was all right for me to be there, she said, "What's he got to say about it? He moved away for twelve years. Irene's been running sun dance here."

I don't recall that I made much response, not wanting an argument, but I thought, *Yeah, she's been squatting in his house, trespassing on his allotment, and trying to steal his sun dance.*

It wasn't Irene who'd brought the sun dance to Ironwood, it was Elmer. He cleared the hilltop and put up the arbor. His dancers and helpers helped with the sweat lodges, dug the fire pit, and poured the concrete for it—and his outfit built the cookshack.

The second day of purification was even worse. Irene and her immediate family, including the young man with the .22 rifle, had ensconced themselves in the cookshack and wouldn't let any of Elmer's crew in. All day, the rest of us toiled on the arbor, finishing the new stringers, and putting the pine boughs in place. Also, there was a lot of just hanging out and discussing the situation. I recall a young guy, a Nakota man I'd met in Santee, recognizing me, and we visited a bit. Since this was to be my fourth year, as an offering of thanks, I'd brought a pickup load of tools, a set of vehicle ramps, and a little modular stereo, and I got these things unloaded. All this, in incredible dry heat—the sun beating down and no shade to be had on the treeless prairie.

By evening, with no working cookshack, and no food forthcoming for the workers, Elmer had had enough. A bunch of us, with him at our head, marched into the cookshack, and he and Irene went at it, head to head. It was the first time I ever saw him raise his voice to a female, but it was all in Lakota, of course, and I couldn't get any of it.

Irene just snarled, got back on her hind legs, and wouldn't budge. We decamped the field, leaving her there, and plans were made to set up a separate tent for the cooks. Elmer always made sure his drummers, singers, security people, and supporters got fed. I remember that evening I suggested to an acquaintance, a sun dancer, that a whole swarm of us go down to the cookshack and wander in by twos and threes until we forced the interlopers out by sheer mass, but no one wanted to take me up on it. I went down there myself, and lo and behold, there she was with some of her kids, smoking pot. I asked her if she wouldn't leave, but of course she just stood there and refused. She asked me if I knew what she was smoking. "Yeah, I know what it is," I said and turned and left.

The next morning, I was pretty excited and nervous because I'd talked to Elmer, and he'd said he'd put me up on the hill. I understood that people had the option of going up for less than four days. I thought I'd spend two days up there, then join in the four days of sun dance. I went up to where Elmer was sitting with his book for the pledgers to record their names and addresses on a little table beside him. He hadn't gotten on the PA yet to tell people to put only four pinches of tobacco in the pipe, "'Cause some o' that tobacco's really strong," as he'd told us in previous years.

Over by the sweat lodges, I was wearing my sun-dancer's skirt and carrying my pipe and bucket of flags and ties. The fires were going full blast, there were others heading in as I approached, and a couple of the senior dancers were there with him. I got close, sat down, and, when a moment presented itself, said, "OK, Elmer, I'm ready to go up." He looked at me kinda funny, seemed to hesitate a moment, then said, "No one's goin' up at this time." Then he pointed across the lodges to where the women were. He grinned and added, "Maybe one o' those women could do it. Put you up."

I just grinned and sort of slunk away.

Later on, one of the men who'd been there during this exchange came by to talk to me. I protested that Elmer had told me I could go up a short time ago. He tried to soften it for me, saying, "He's getting old and a little forgetful."

I'd gone back to my camp and changed back to regular work clothes, feeling terrible and trying to stifle my resentment. That crack about the women had really stung, though. I'd been in the category of men who couldn't make it through a couple of his hotter sweats, and the talk about wearing a dress was never followed through on, but for some reason that day's crack had hurt, when the former had never really bothered me.

But now I felt it was time for me to get in line to pledge. I got in line with my *canunpa*, which had been loaded for *hanble-chiya*, and waited, looking around. There were a lot of people around us, and the atmosphere was looser and wilder than I'd ever felt it at Santee. The presence of Irene and her bunch plus strangers was like loud white noise in the background. There was a group of Indians, all guys, camped a little ways uphill from where Elmer had his tipi and chair set up, looking down on us in more ways than one, kinda snickering.

By the time I was in line to sign, a couple of these guys had passed through Elmer's area there, and when he went to get his long-nosed lighter to light my pipe, it was gone. Other things, including a pair of pliers and other small items, were disappearing. We had to scare up a box of matches for my pipe, and the old man was getting mad by then. Next, I went to help him set up the PA and had to go find another pair of pliers. When he directed me to twist a certain dial to get the system powered up, I didn't listen and tried another switch that I thought would do it. No luck. Someone else came up and followed his advice, and then we had a working PA. I sort of had to slink away again, since his refusal earlier wasn't helping me get a good attitude going.

That morning, or the rest of it, anyway, I busied myself helping put up the last of the pine boughs over the rest area where the dancers would take their breaks. This was enclosed with a wall on the western side, as well, so it took extra work. Someone was providing Gatorade for the workers, and I'd put away a couple of pints by noon. The lunch break was called, and I sat down to eat with the others in the arbor. About halfway through my sandwich and chips, I noticed something odd. I'd stopped sweating. I'd been about soaked through by ten, as hot as it was, but now my skin was clammy. I was starting to feel bad—sick, in fact—and when I stood up after lunch, a wave of nausea hit me. I walked away from the arbor, and when I got to the little road that separated Elmer's tipi from the gang uphill, I heaved up everything I'd eaten, and a lot of Gatorade too. One of the uphill thieves saw me and started laughing at me. That was my last straw. I was dizzy, light-headed, and I knew I had to get out of the sun right away, since I'd (accurately) self-diagnosed a case of heat stroke. I staggered over to my pickup, drove over to

Norman and Shannon's, knocked at the door, explained myself, got permission, and rolled myself up in a blanket in their little added-on TV room, with the big air conditioner. Stayed there all night without eating, barely conscious, and most of the next day, which was tree day.

CHAPTER 14

Seven-Year Hiatus

I'D RECOVERED ENOUGH TO DRIVE BACK OUT TO IRONWOOD ON the evening of the fourth day. I managed to make my way back up to the arbor, just as the sun-dance tree was set upright and placed in its pit. I watched from outside the circle in a sort of angry, dazed stupor, feeling sick in heart and body. I turned away without speaking to anyone and walked back to my vehicle. Earlier on the day I'd gotten sick, I'd given away some of the things I'd planned to save for *wopila* after sun dance. I seem to recall throwing my flags and ties in the sweat-lodge fire at some point, since it was obvious they weren't going to be used, and there was no point in keeping them. I drove slowly back to Norman's, spent the night again on the back room floor, and drove back to Nebraska the next morning. It was seven years before I saw Elmer again.

I have to admit I was very bitter about not being able to finish my fourth year. At first, I blamed everyone but myself: Elmer, for trading me out of my favorite jacket, for putting up with Gilli's abuse, and for changing his mind about putting me up on the hill; Irene for her static and intimidation; and Patti, for talking me into putting the *canunpa* I'd been gifted for my first sun dance out on the hill. And the thievin' Injuns of Rosebud.

I'd slipped back into the habit of smoking grass, or *pegi*, as it's called in NDN country. The humiliating fact that I was thinking more of the fourth set of scars I'd have than I was of dedicating my suffering to the people so that they might live didn't dawn on me until long afterward. I'd gotten rid of all the stuff I'd harvested at Santee, but in the summer of 2000, I'd picked some roadside weed that looked promising, and I'd been smoking that. Not that I'd brought any with me or shared in the offering from Irene in the cookshack, since I had too much respect for the old man for that, as well as too much apprehension of what the spirits might do to me or to a loved one. But I wish I hadn't slid back.

Later on, during my third year away, I even got back into drinking. My family all liked a few glasses of wine with dinner, and I was often present. I began to miss the conviviality, so in the fall of 2005, I started off with a bottle of white. It ended up costing me greatly.

I was living in a remote cabin in northeastern Iowa at the time. I'd gotten two other shih tzus, and they were my constant companions. I was really pushing myself the last days I was there, putting in a homemade heat shield on the wall and a ceramic tile floor guard for the new woodstove. Winter was coming on, and I needed to have the insurance man come to inspect it all, so as to be able to buy a policy before heading back to Nebraska, since I had no woodpile.

Well, he came, took some pictures, and told me it looked OK and that the insurance forms would be ready to sign on my way out of town. I'd had to stay up most of the night, packing and doing the stove work, so I shouldn't have tried to drive as far as I did the next day. After signing the forms, I gassed up my vehicle and headed west. About halfway to my first night's lodgings, gray, foggy weather closed in. In the midst of this, what should I see but an owl flying from left to right, directly across my path. This I knew was a sign from the spirits to be feared, and I was correct, very much so. Since beginning to pray and trying to walk the good red road back in 1986, I'd had owls come to me, and each one had presaged a death. And indeed, one of my little dogs slipped out of my motel room after I'd left to bring in a load of clothes after dark. She ran across the road, and when I called to her, in a panic, crossed back and was killed right in front of me by a car that never even slowed down. At least she was killed instantly. Being so tired, I'd neglected to shut the door completely. I hadn't thought any of them would leave, with a fresh, fragrant pizza in the room, but she did.

It completely did me in. I spent the rest of the night—after I'd picked up her body, wrapped it in a towel, and put it in the truck's toolbox—howling and crying my eyes out. One woman, who'd been behind the vehicle that hit, actually came to my room, knocked on the door, and said she'd seen the whole thing and gave me a big hug, but I was inconsolable. I don't blame the owl, or the spirits, or Patti for talking me into putting my pipe up out on the hill (which made me believe that my commitment to Elmer's altar was broken), or even the driver. I did it with my drinking. I'd been warned about exactly this kind of thing happening to those who don't respect the pipe and the old ways, and I didn't listen.

This brings to mind a happening at my second sun dance in Santee, the year before I went to live there and work with Grandpa. As the pledgers were tying on their flags, ties, and ropes, I made the unintentional mistake of stepping over one of the branches of the tree. I knew it was a bad thing to have done. I'd been warned against it, just as I'd been warned against drugs and alcohol and against crossing the east gate. The next afternoon, during a long dance round, the arch of the foot I'd stepped over with became elevated. Not broken, just stretched up out of position. I'd had this happen before after hard work with a shovel, and it was really painful. Nonetheless, I kept on dancing.

The spirits demand respect, once their aid had been sought, and, as Elmer told us, "The spirits, they're kinda particular."

Well, I was heartbroken over the loss of my dog, but I still wouldn't pay heed. Kept on drinking. Had dinners with my relatives, had wine with my supper at home, and by the winter of 2008, I had somehow begun to repeatedly break my left little toe. I lost count of how many times I stubbed it hard enough to break it. Nothing the docs can do with such a small break, either. It has to mend on its own, and each time it does it gets more rough and uneven. I don't think this started until after I'd begun to drink at home and started making wine. I had a press, a big glass carboy, and everything. That year, I lost a big batch to a mold and quit the making, but kept on drinking.

But to backtrack a bit, in the spring of 2006, just as I was about to head back to the little cabin in Iowa that I'd worked so hard to set up the previous fall, and the single-wide trailer I planned to use as storage, and as a recording studio, I got a call from Decorah. Seems that the Friday of the full moon just before the vernal equinox, somebody set fire to the trailer. That set me back a bit, but not as hard as the following Monday when I got another call, this time from an Iowa state fire marshal, telling me that whoever it was had come back Saturday night and finished the job by burning down the cabin. "They must have come in Saturday night after we'd left and done it then," he told me. I was stunned. Nothing was going right.

Now it came clear to me why getting the insurance in place had seemed so urgent. No question but it was arson. When I finally did get back there, in late May, I had an interview with the police, who had no leads, and with the realtor who'd sold me the property. He was a local resident and said it might have been some poacher who'd been jacking deer out of the adjacent state park. Although the insurance company and the fire marshal's office were each offering substantial rewards, no one knows who did it. Someone who didn't want me there—but I knew practically no one in the area, aside from a few shopkeepers, and certainly didn't have any enemies. Anyhow, the insurance company paid up without a quibble, so I had a tidy sum—less about a grand or so for cleanup costs—to tool around the Upper Midwest on. I'd been feeling a pull up there.

At the cabin site, I saw firsthand how a hot fire can reduce cast iron to the consistency of cardboard and sheet metal, as in a stove or fridge, to the level of paper. It was also the first time I ever felt compelled to arm myself with deadly force. I stopped in at a little reenactment outfitters, bought a .45 cap-and-ball six-shooter, and a Kirst Konverter that allowed it to fire black-powder loads in cartridges. There was no federal law against conversion weapons then, and black powder arms aren't classed as firearms, anyway, so I was free to strap on a hogleg the day I bought it, head out to the site of my former cabin in the woods, and survey the results.

Well, I was done with Iowa. I headed north to Minnesota and discovered a little town on the upper Mississippi called Red Wing. At first, I stayed in an apartment, thinking I'd enroll in the instrument-making course at the state technical college. The next year, I found a little property on the opposite side of town with a little bungalow-style house on it that I was able to purchase with the insurance money. It took quite a bit of work to make it habitable; the renovations weren't complete 'til 2010.

But in the fall of 2008, I happened to see a poster for the "All Relatives Have Come Home" Dakota homecoming powwow in a river town south of Red Wing. So I went and had a fairly good time.

I didn't tell anyone there I'd been a sun dancer, and there was no one there I knew. I did talk with one older lady a bit about how I'd been indirectly involved with the restoration of some tribal remains of the Abenaki during my time in Vermont by house-sitting for a couple who were the main force behind the repatriation. But while scoping out the vendors, I noticed one couples' stand—with a *canunpa* for sale. I bought several other items elsewhere first, beads and whatnot, but somehow kept finding myself drawn back to that one booth.

At last, I stopped there and asked to see the pipe. The man running it had noticed my repeated reconnoiterings and said, "It's calling to you." And it did indeed seem to be. In the end, I bought it. He started telling me how the stem should never be put together with the bowl until one was ready to pray. I thanked him and told him I already knew the basics of how to handle a *canunpa*, and we shook hands.

Since I was still drinking a glass or two of wine with my dinner, I knew better than to start using it. I got some red felt, a nice little beaded pipe bag from Thunder Clan, the local NDN store in Red Wing, put some sage with it, and kept it in a little back room at the bungalow, where the dogs were not allowed. I wondered why I was doing all this and why I'd gotten it in the first place, but there it was.

During the seven years away, I kept making my monthly ceremony ties, plus some special strings for help and/or emergency situations, and I had quite a big bag of old ones and no way to properly dispose of them, since I had no access to a sweat-lodge fire. I had considered putting up a little *inipi* in the woods back of my house in Nebraska, but I had no eagle feather for the staff, plus the only time I'd tried to pour sweat, I'd poured too fast, cracked the grandfathers, and lightly scalded the two guys who'd come late to monthly ceremony in Santee. Elmer had told me to do it for these latecomers, saying, "You could do it for them; you a sun dancer." But he'd had a kind of mocking look in his eye as he'd said it. The actual pouring, with the accompanying songs, was something I'd never been able to observe. I'd heard the songs and joined in on the choruses I was sure of, but it's not possible to see in total darkness.

Well, the year began to wear on. The holidays were approaching, so I closed up the little bungalow, gathered up the pipe, my dogs, and instruments and headed back to Nebraska. I'd gotten another shih tzu, a male puppy, soon after I'd gotten back in late 2005. Not so much to replace the one who was killed but because having only two with me when I'd been used to three was a constant reminder of the unhappy event. This new guy I named Buddy, and he's lived up to his name. Always eager for a run, ready to play or cuddle up, and he got Belle, the female I'd gotten when I first left Santee, pregnant. She had a litter of six, of which only three survived.

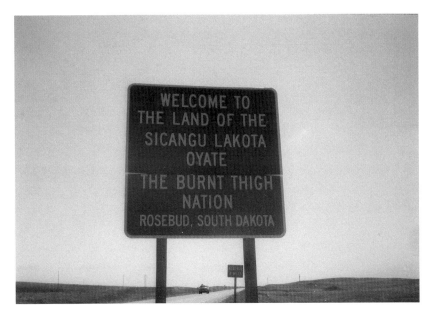

Reservation entrance

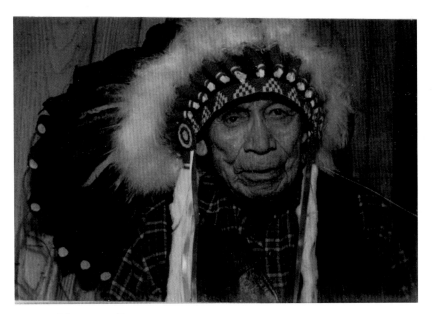

Elmer Norbert Running

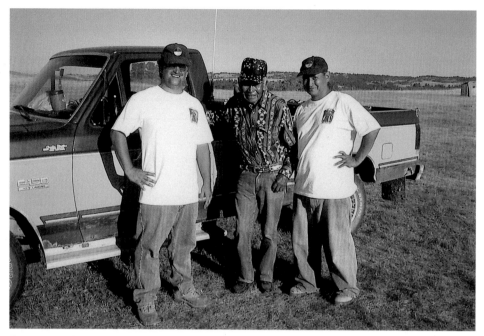

PATRICK, GRANDPA, SUNDANCER

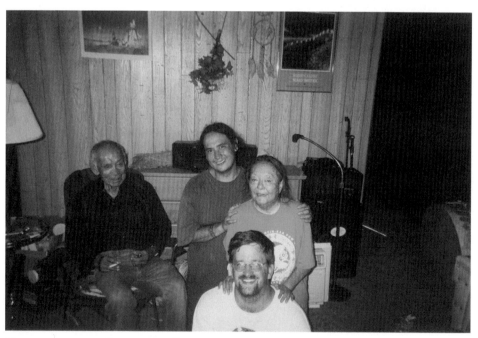

GRANDPA WITH GRANDMA DAR AND DANCERS

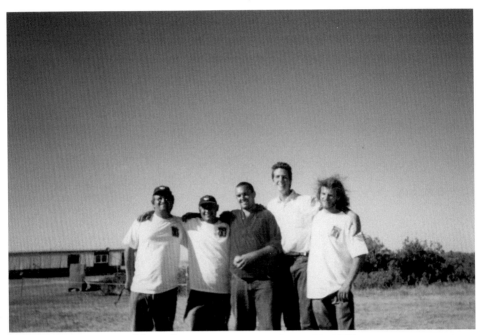

SUNDANCERS, WITH MIKE JAGOD SECOND FROM THE LEFT

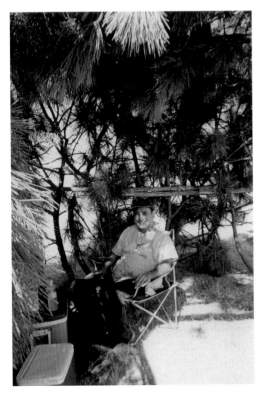

MIKE JAGOD IN THE SHADEARBOR

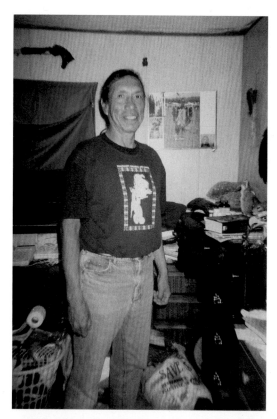

GILLI

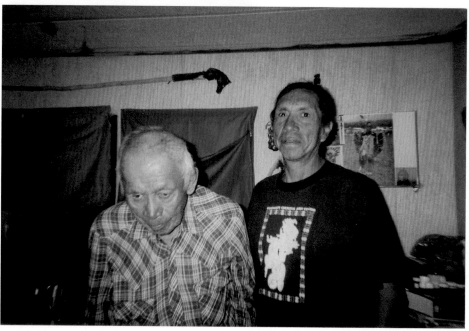

GRANDPA AND GILLI

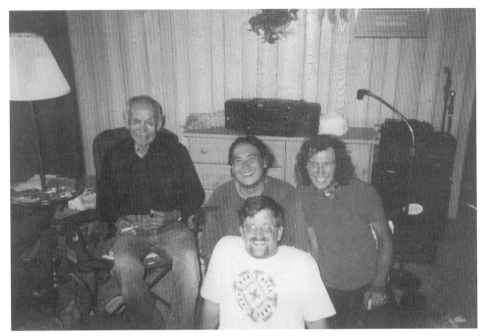

GRANDPA WITH SUNDANCERS AND CAMP CRIER, JASON KOLBO (RED SHIRT)

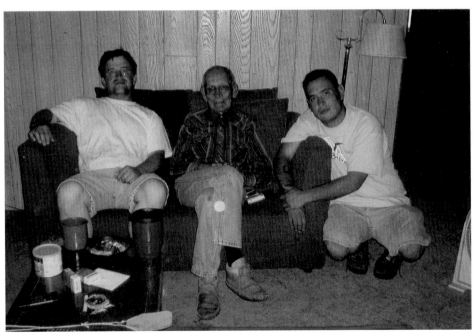

: PATRICK, GRANDPA, AND MIKE JAGOD

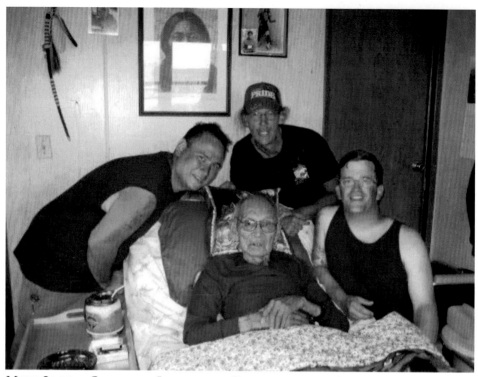

MIKE JAGOD, GRANDPA, JASON, AND PATRICK

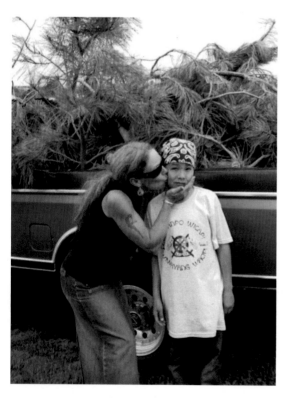

GWEN AND SAGE

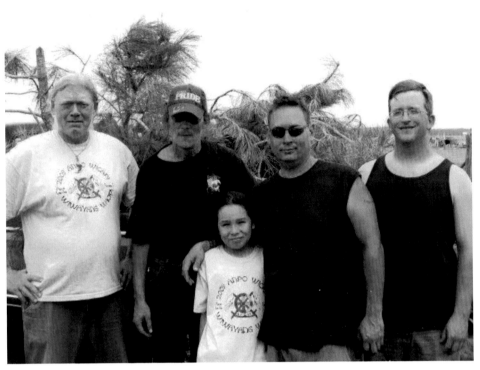

THE AUTHOR, JASON, SAGE, MIKE, AND PATRICK

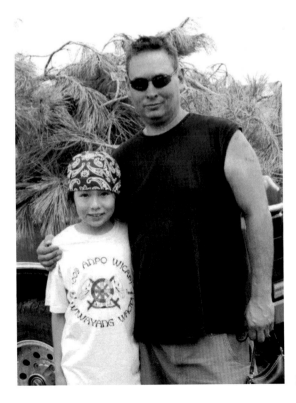

SAGE AND MIKE

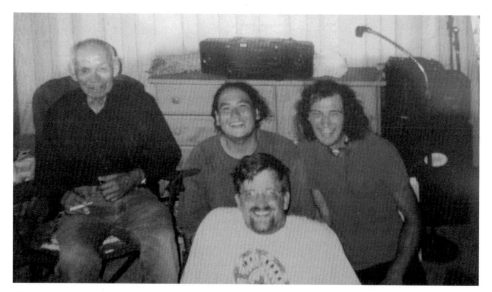

Grandpa, Don, and Jason

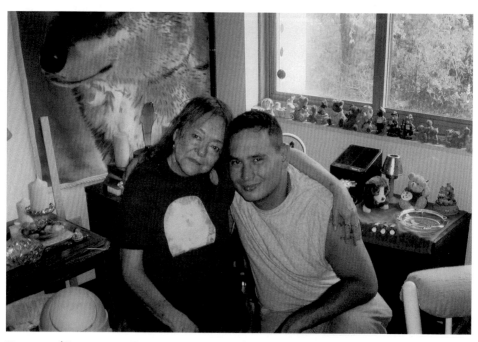

Bozhoo (Grandma Darlene Jackson) with Mike Jagod

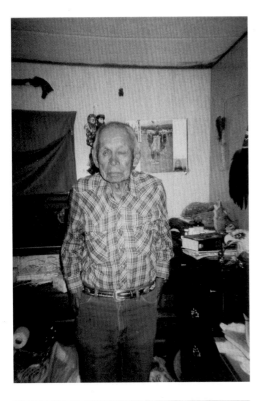

GRANDPA IN HIS BEDROOM, WITH
PORTRAIT OF HIMSELF IN TRADI-
TIONAL DANCER'S REGALIA

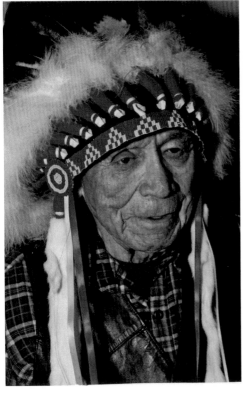

GRANDPA IN HIS EAGLE-FEATHER
HEADDRESS, CIRCA 2000

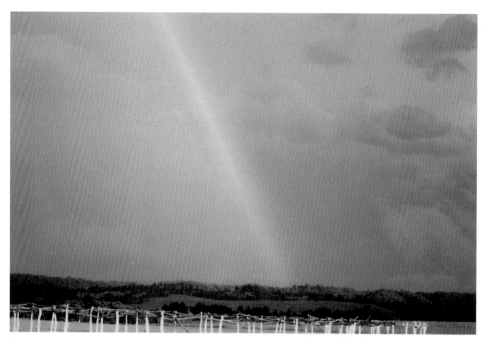

Rainbow over Sundance arbor, Rosebad

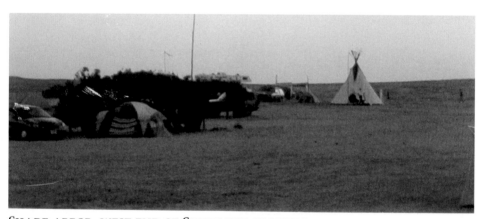

Shade arbor, west end of Sundance grounds

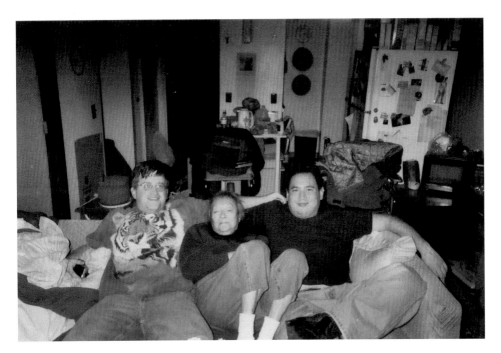

Bozhoo with Sundancers

PART 4
Rosebud, 2008–09

Chapter 15

Answering the Call

I HAD SOME HELP FINDING GOOD HOMES FOR THE TWO MALE pups when they were old enough and kept the white-and-ginger female, Lizzie. Then I had Buddy fixed. We all passed the winter in Nebraska and went up to Minnesota again in 2008—but that was not only the year of the economic meltdown and the big bridge collapse in Minneapolis, but it rained the whole summer; I couldn't get much done. Again overwintering in Nebraska, in February of 2009, something woke me up in the small hours one morning. It was about two thirty, and I was startled by a loud, heavy-sounding pounding on the floor of the room above my bedroom: *Wham-wham-wham-wham-wham.*

I lay in bed, somewhat dazed, wondering what it could be. I began to recognize it. *Oh yeah*, I thought. *That's the same sound the rawhide rattles used to make in ceremony when the spirits pick them up and pound them on the floor, and they flash as if tiny lightnings were inside 'em.* Anyone who has ever heard it would not soon forget. I wondered what was happening and drifted back to sleep. Soon it came again. Same tangible impact in the house, same rapid-fire beat. Later, when I'd had time to reflect on things, I realized that the presence of a *canunpa* was the key to their entrance. I kept my ties and sage—and, of course, the pipe—in a little prayer room upstairs.

When I went up there the next morning, I found two little nails that had held the plywood panel in place on the wall that led to the open airspace under the roof had been pounded out of the wood and lay on the shelf beneath. I knew the spirits were calling me back to help out and to finish my fourth year.

So that June, I put the critters into boarding and headed back up to South Dakota. I was leaving early, as I intended to attend the Rainbow Family Fourth of July gathering, then head back to Red Wing until it was nearly time for purification. I also planned to do some good for some of the other attendees by bringing a humongous amount of food and utensils and by and setting up a small kitchen. I even saw a brilliant rainbow in the eastern sky one evening a day or two before I left.

Getting back up to Rosebud was no problem, but I had to ask directions to Elmer's. He wasn't at Norman and Shannon's or at his old outfit in Ironwood. He was a mile or less west of there, in the same old beat-up double-wide at the bottom of a steep hill. Well set up on level ground, across a fence line from a cattle rancher who was leasing part of Elmer's allotment. The new ceremony house was south of the trailer, with the sun-dance grounds a few hundred yards east of it and the sweat lodges between them.

When I got there, he didn't know me. Gilli was still there, ostensibly taking care of him, but there was an air of general neglect. The water wasn't hooked up too well; there was no drainage from the trailer. One had to use an outhouse in all weather. I also noticed that many of the fine things were gone from the old man's bedroom—tokens of gratitude with which he'd been gifted over many years. His chainsaw was on a shelf in his bedroom, and there was a lock and hasp on the door to it.

I was let in by Gilli, and Elmer came up to the living room and introduced himself with a big warm smile. "I'm Elmer."

I introduced myself and told him I'd come to help out and to sun dance.

"You the first one to come this year," he said, shaking my hand.

I mentioned to Gilli later that I didn't think he'd recognized me. Elmer was, if possible, even thinner than when I'd known him in Santee and a little more stooped. But he still seemed his usual happy self. I think it was then that I noticed the resemblance of his expression to that of the Dalai Lama's. He seemed a bit downcast when I told him I wasn't staying on just then but that I'd be back later on in time to help out for sun dance. I did lay some cigarettes on them both and a whole bunch of discount steaks and burgers I'd bought frozen just before I left, forgetting the times he'd warned us against "the chemicals they're puttin' in that cow meat."

The next thing he said, though, was, "You could sleep right there," pointing to the old couch in the living room. How many people would take in people they apparently didn't know and let them sleep in their homes, without being asked? Not very many, nowadays. Having devoured all the Native resources it could get to, not just once but many times, postcolonial Euro-America has wantonly begun devouring and laying waste to itself.

I recall the incident at the Columbine High School that took place in 1999 while I was staying with Pete, Elmer, and Patti in Santee. We were all watching the afternoon news, kinda quietly horrified, like everyone else, when Patti said, "There's gonna be more of that."

It's too bad most Americans have absolutely no sense of their own history, and what most do know of it has been so watered down and whitewashed that they have no conception of the massive theft, betrayal, and nearly total genocide that took place so modern America could exist. I think I know what Patti meant and why there's going to be more incidents like the Columbine shooting. What goes around, comes back around.

For over six hundred years now, Native people have had to watch while their leaders have been either seduced, suborned, or exterminated; their customs and religion vilified, ridiculed, and outlawed; and their children forcibly turned to the ways of an alien invader, often so brutalized in the process they couldn't function well in either their own fragmented tribes or the conformist masses of white society. Millions of Native families have been destroyed by alcohol, disease, forced displacement, and racist intolerance. Their surviving children, as they grew up, became so crazy from confusion, racism, rage, and despair they contribute to the disintegration. Now it's the white people's turn. Nothing can stop it.

But Grandpa was never one to give up hope. "Don't think about you'self," he'd say. "Just think about the people. 'Cause what we need is good health and help." That's what he told us to pray for, and "not just for the Indian people, but all the people in this world."

I stayed around all that day, loaded up their little freezer with my beef offerings, emptied the drain bucket from under the kitchen sink, and did what else I could. I hooked up my home-made camper (not the 1995 Chev I'd had in Santee, but a newer one by Ford, almost the same vehicle, what they call a cube van) to the power pole by the cookshack and stayed one night. Said good-bye the next morning, shook hands, and told them I'd be back after the Rainbow Gathering.

On the way to the gathering, which was way north in Wyoming that year, I got to thinking I wanted to get a drum so I could sit in on the drum circle. I decided I'd try to find a little Indian store somewhere. I'd had a good trip so far. This was about the second day out from Rosebud. On the first day, I'd stopped at a big patch of sage that was growing along the high-way. I'd been on the lookout for some, but none of the growths I'd spotted contained plants tall enough to harvest. This one did. In fact, there was already another carload of folks picking it when I zoomed past. I turned around and chatted a bit with them, and one guy offered me some tobacco as an offering to the plants. I thanked him and told them I'd already made one discreetly, on my way across the highway. They seemed mostly friendly, but one of the men was wary of me. I could sense his reserve, and I decided it was a case of his being a little too careful. I'm a large man, and sometimes I tend to intimidate without even being aware of it.

Anyway, I got my bundle and put it on the dashboard to dry. I also stopped at the Museum of the Fur Trade, just outside of Chadron, and got some cool repro trade beads for my crafting. I saw a sign that indicated the way up to Whiteclay, since I was now south of where I'd left Rosebud, but there was no way I was heading through that awful place.

Whiteclay, Nebraska's enduring shame, where the state refuses to enforce its own liquor laws, allows on-premises and public consumption of alcohol and is located just over the state line from Pine Ridge, South Dakota. Take away everything from a people, not just once but many times, and then allow them access to unregulated alcohol. From a distance, the aim of the establishment is crystal clear: We hope to provide you the means to finish yourselves off so we don't have to. Plus, some white men are getting rich off the despair and continuing genocide of the Oglala. I have myself called the Nebraska Liquor Control Commission and left messages for the personnel involved in enforcement and never got a single return call.

Pine Ridge, formerly the Red Cloud Indian Agency. Pine Ridge, where shadow agents from the FBI's Counterintelligence Program (COINTELPRO) shipped in military-grade weapons to the corrupt tribal council's goons. Pine Ridge, where the FBI murdered Anna Mae Aquash and cut off her hands "for identification." Pine Ridge, where a firefight between FBI agents and AIM left two agents and one Lakota man dead—and resulted in the railroading of Leonard Peltier into two consecutive life terms for murders he didn't commit. Pine Ridge, this country's gulag, America's everlasting shame. The Red Shirt Table district of Pine Ridge, where the Canadian firm Cameco's uranium mining leach-water spills have contaminated the groundwater and are, just like the man said in the movie *Thunderheart*, "turning this reservation into a dead zone."

So I continued west most of that day, until I came to the little town of Douglas, Wyoming. Still looking for a drum, but not knowing the layout, I first scouted a little strip mall with a thrift store, but no luck. Then I pulled the van into the parking lot of a large café. Once inside, I took a seat and asked the waitress if she knew of any places in town that sold Indian-made goods. "Well, there's Morningstar's," she said. "That's in town, and the lady who owns it is sitting right over there." Indeed, there was a Native-looking lady of some advanced years sitting with a friend, smoking and drinking coffee. I introduced myself and told her I was after a drum. "I closed the shop last year," she told me, "but I do have one old drum, with no stick, that I could sell."

"Any old beads? Chevrons, maybe?" I asked after thanking her.

"Yes, I have some chevrons and some odds and ends of stock left from the store, but I'll have to go home and get them."

She proceeded to direct me to a little riverside campground right in the middle of town, where I could park overnight. She said she'd meet me there later on in the evening.

The park turned out to be everything she said and more. There were even showers with free hot water for the use of overnight guests. There was a minimal camping fee, on the honor system. So I put my money in the little envelope in the box by the men's-room door and made some supper while I waited for her.

When she arrived, a little after seven, we sat down and did some dealing. She had a nice little hand drum, a large strand of old chevron beads, and a big bag of miscellaneous glass and trade beads. We came to a fair price for the lot, and then we had a talk. I told her about my visit to Elmer, whom she'd heard of, but when I told her, "The old man's having to sleep with his chainsaw in his bedroom; that told me all I needed to know," she snorted in disgust.

She said she was of Cherokee descent and that her father had given her her name, since she'd been born just before sunrise, when only the morning star was in the sky. I told of not knowing much about my own miniscule Native heritage until I'd been invited by a friend to a powwow in Connecticut in 1986—and beginning to have some interesting experiences after I'd begun praying in the Indian way. Centering first around the drum, then later on seeing things on the powwow grounds, then later in the sky.

Chapter 16

An Interlude at the Rainbow Gathering

I T SEEMED TO BE ENOUGH TO CONVINCE HER OF MY SINCERITY. When I told her that I really wanted to get back to Rosebud to complete my fourth year as soon as the Rainbow Gathering was over, but that I was nervous about the alcohol, since I knew I'd really have to put it down for good and all, she exclaimed, "Come back to the good red road, brother."

"I'm afraid of what could happen if I'm not strong enough to let it go," I told her. "It's brought down better men than me."

She grabbed me in a fierce bear hug and said, "Don't be afraid." Again and again, those words have come back to me.

She advised me against going to the Rainbow Gathering, saying she'd had a friend who'd had a terrible experience there, but I was all set for one last go-round. I did finish off one bottle of wine that evening, with supper, but that was it. I haven't had a drop since.

The gathering itself is just a blur to me now. I was stopped and searched by the cops, mostly Park Service and State, and had to wait while they searched the van. They lied—said their dope-sniffing dog had "alerted" while it was in back of the camper, and so conveniently out of my sight. They kept me there for three hours, until it was dark, and found nothing. The next day I set up my little kitchen, camped with a bunch of nouveau hippies, and didn't trip and go off the deep end as I'd done at previous gatherings. In fact, I think I did some good and hopefully redeemed some of that negative karma, which was why I needed to go there in the first place.

I maintained a large, communal trench latrine, with considerable help, and fed a lotta kids and some older folks. The Forest Service was as obnoxious as they could possibly be, sending out patrols, hassling people, and checking to make sure fire regulations were being observed at all hours. It was a pretty wild ride; I never got to drum at the drum circle—spent all my time digging shitters, cooking and washing up and trying to keep a sanitary kitchen, begging toilet paper, and talking people down who'd gotten too high. Whew. I've been told I have a tendency to overplay my responsibilities sometimes.

But all in all, I had a good time and even found a helper to come along and do some of the work, or so I thought. He called himself White Hawk, and he was one of the young'uns who'd camped close to where I set up the kitchen. He said he'd been in a bad communal situation before coming to the gathering. He worked with a bunch on a farm, who barely fed him enough, and he had no help from his family of origin. But he could play the flute well, and he used it to cool things out. But I immediately had a feeling that he was work shy. I sort of took a shine to him and felt sorry for him too.

He was the one who told me I'd missed the big show at Monkeytown, which was what I'd called our little kitchen and camp area. A young lady had come into camp and took her top off after a bit. She said it was the first camp she'd come to where she wasn't hassled to do so, so we got the glory. Made me feel good about the quality of the people who'd been attracted to my outfit, though.

Now, all this was taking place in alpine meadows and woods at around eleven thousand feet. It's hard to get water boiling for coffee (or anything else) at such an elevation. Also, at that altitude, the only firewood is lodgepole pine, and the smoke is dense, pitchy, and not good to breathe. Plus, altitude sickness was a real, if sporadic, problem. I was glad I had my allergy inhalers and antihistamines, since I had to get a couple of folks breathing again when they'd had too much. Well, the Forest Service finally ousted us by setting a little fire off somewhere and then announcing, "Mandatory fire evacuation." You could see how much they enjoyed abusing their official status. They were recorded doing this by someone on hand with a smartphone, so who needs the cops?

I was still having a good time, but it was time to start thinking about getting myself in the proper frame of mind for sun dance: less chaotic, more prayerful. I had, in fact, been a pretty good scout, if I do say so myself—no psychedelic adventures, no drinking, and no chasing the *wincincalas*. I worked hard for the people.

During the last few days, as people left and trusted the cleanup crews to dismantle and recycle their remains, various campsites were deserted, and the contents became fair game for whoever got there first. I got a beautiful tie-dye print, a little antler pipe, and some new camp chairs. Some thoughtful souls even scooped out the ashes from their fire pit and left them in a container at the latrine. Finally, however, we were all given the bum's rush. The latrine walls (made of bark and tarp) were taken down, the pits ashed and covered with earth, the big tarp, tents, and kitchen supplies packed up, and we were on the long, downhill hike to the parking area.

I couldn't help but notice, though, that when the hard work of camp-busting came around, White Hawk was nowhere to be found. He must have been watching, though, because when the youngsters and I began to head out into the meadow, he turned up and took a share of the burden. I wanted badly to grab a set of abandoned lodgepoles from where some folks had been camping in tipis, but he talked me out of it each time I brought it up. I only let him because I was too tired to argue and, given the construction of the box portion of my vehicle, it would have been hard to lash them on top. I did manage to score two four-inch-diameter, ten-foot bamboo poles that I planned on making into a flute or a set of bass panpipes.

As expected, the higher parking area was chaos. Some folks were staying on to help with the cleanup; some were simply stranded, having hitched a ride in and then unable to find one out. While I was waiting for a young man who'd been a camper at Monkeytown to show up so we could depart, a very disoriented-looking young lady wandered up right up to the fire where I was chatting with a fellow who'd set up a kitchen for the cleaners and refugees.

She seemed distracted, rather disheveled (as were we all), but talking in a strange sort of incoherent "meemblings." We all got up and sort of tried to help. She was obviously distressed and trying to communicate. After a cup of coffee and some trail mix, she calmed down and explained she needed a ride to Minneapolis, which was where our party was bound. Can't recall her name, but she was black Irish and never lost that somewhat fey quality the whole time we traveled.

We passed some pretty desperate folks on the lower approaches to the forest. We'd picked up another young man, a latecomer to Monkeytown, plus another who was heading out to the Twin Cities. With five of us in all, I had to tell all the other hitchers we were full up. The evening main-circle feeds had gotten a bit slender the last couple of days at the gathering, so I stopped at a place I'd gassed up at on the way in—a big truck stop right across a side road from an ice-cream parlor. Since I had the means, I told everyone to get what they wanted, it was on me. We'd come to the right place. We got big sugar cones topped with huge scoops of homemade-style ice cream.

"Wow! That ain't no main-circle portion!" exclaimed the late-comer to a round of laughs. Even the Irish girl clapped her hands with delight. We were a bunch of happy campers as we headed off into the sunset of the Golden West.

That evening, we stopped at a remote campground in southern Wyoming. We must have left early in the day because I recall that after we set up camp, I slept out in a blanket, surrounded by the large bundles of sage we'd picked on the way, plus the four buffalo skulls I bought during our noon stop in a little town for sun dance. We made a fair piece of distance that day, despite the stops, and had a nice dinner by the campfire we erected a wall of stones around; we'd had to. We were on the shore of a dry lake bed, across which the wind off the Rockies blew constantly. The whole area was still up in the foothills, and I recall wishing I could stay there longer. Soon after occupying our site, White Hawk and I went out on a firewood hunt, and we'd both spotted a big vulture feather at the same time. It was like it was waiting there, and since I was a bit closer, I claimed it. I pulled out a little hair to leave in return. That's one thing I've learned of the Indian ways; you don't just find and take.

But it was the next day, when we went back through Douglas, Wyoming, that things got weird with White Hawk. I'd warned him and the others to be discreet about their consumption of pot in my vehicle. It was really important to me that I be able to get back to Rosebud in time to help out and finish my fourth year, even though it had been so long. Those spirits, pounding on the floor upstairs that night, had left a big impression. Plus, on my way up to the gathering, as I'd crossed the Continental Divide, I'd pulled off onto a scenic overlook, and there, like it was waiting for me, was the almost-fresh wing of some large raptor, practically intact. All it needed was a few days with salt on the fleshy parts, to be ready for use as a dance-fan. At first I thought it was the wing of a golden eagle, but it turned out to be buzzard. Nonetheless, I was pretty happy to have it.

So White Hawk was traveling with me to the Twin Cities. He'd agreed to stay on as a sort of a helper, with me as straw boss. I was feeding him, trying to pay him what I thought I could afford, since neither of us wanted a formal employer-employee deal. It probably wasn't up to minimum wage, but it was still a damn sight better than he'd been doing on the communal farm—where, he told me, he'd been losing weight. So we parked on the main drag in Douglas, and he stayed in the vehicle while I went across the street to check out an antique shop. Correction: We went into a little antique shop across the street, and lo and behold, there was a silver-plated flute, his instrument. He used most of what I'd paid him so far to buy it and went back to the van. I went into the next store and was enjoying the various jumbles of stuff; it was my kind of place, stuff piled on shelves up to the ceilings, all kinds of things. To me, it's hunting. I'd picked out a set of pronghorn antelope antlers, and I was looking at something else, when a policeman walked up to me and asked if I was the owner of the white van across the way.

I told him yes.

He said there was a situation, and he'd have to ask me to accompany him back to the vehicle.

Wondering what in hell was going on, I accompanied him along the block, but he refused to let me cross the street. He wanted me to stay away from the scene with White Hawk.

There were several officers, one lady cop, going through the front of the van. The Irish girl and the young dude were sitting on the curb, and the Hawk was sitting on a bench next to a cop a little ways away, looking scared. Turns out, he'd completely ignored my instructions and pulled out his little glass pipe from the purple Seagram's bag and was busily scraping up a bowl of resin when the lady traffic cop came along and saw him. This I didn't find out 'til later—for who should come up to where the cop and I were waiting but Morningstar.

She had a very determined look as she asked the young cop with me, "What's going on?"

I thought the officer was going to pee his pants as he replied, in a very fast and nervous-sounding voice, very unlike the one he'd used to address me, "Now just take it easy, Morningstar. We're not arresting this one. It's the guy in the vehicle we're looking at, no reason to get excited," and so on. In a word, he backed down like a pup in a pack who'd just pissed off the alpha female. It was truly awesome. By now, a plainclothes detective had joined our merry throng, just hanging back at the end of the block, watching. Like I say, I'd rather go a day without food or water than piss off a Cherokee grandma. Those Tsalagi (Cherokee), they keep on coming into it with me.

Anyway, Morningstar took me across the street to deal with the situation, and I was sat down on the sidewalk bench next to White Hawk while the cops once again searched the van, finding nothing. I forced myself to remain calm, despite the fact that I was fairly exercised at him, and when the cop who was explaining it all to me mentioned the penalties for possession to him, and he started back-sassing her, and one of the older guy cops shouted him down, ending with, "Be like this guy here! He's bein' polite!"

Since they'd found nothing, they had to let us go, but not before giving the Hawk a ticket for possession of paraphernalia, with a court date. I'd made arrangements with Morningstar to meet with her at the location of her old store to get some Native music on CD for the trip east. When we got there, she lit into him, saying, "He's a sun dancer—he's got to finish his fourth year." Then, turning to me, she said, "You should just let him go on down the road his own way. He's a pothead, and he's just gonna drag you down."

She was right too; the few extra bottles of wine I'd had with me, which I'd thought I'd left behind for the cleanup crews at the gathering, were still on board. He'd scrounged them without telling me. I asked Morningstar to get rid of it for me and began handing the bottles to her.

"What am I gonna do with it?" she protested.

"Please take it off me," I pleaded. "Give it to some of your friends who still do drink."

"OK," she said, reluctantly grabbing hold of them. Despite the fact that White Hawk did make several material contributions, before, during, and after sun dance, I later had reason to wish I'd followed her advice.

We had a fairly uneventful time after that, except for the time we stopped in Rapid City, South Dakota. I wanted to go to the Prairie Edge Trading Co. & Galleries to get a few more things for sun dance and for myself. But the two passengers were impatient to get back to Minneapolis: "Karl's going shopping again," they complained and threatened to continue on their own if I didn't get with it. I spent a little time at the Edge but soon got back on the road. At one point, I could swear I heard them giving each other a vivid account of my shortcomings as they were sitting right behind me in the back of the van. Sorry. I've had freedom from employment for long enough that I forget that others have to be at work on time.

It was late the next night when I dropped them off in their neighborhood in Minneapolis and headed down to Red Wing. Finding my way through the maze of the Twin Cities' freeways and state highways was a chore, but luckily I'd had the bene-fit of a few prior visits, mostly to Grandma Darlene's. That was little help, however, since the area I was partly familiar with was under extensive construction. I was forced to detour and ended up in the middle of downtown Minneapolis, far from where I needed to be and unable to find my way out. I had to stop twice for directions but at last got headed south—and an hour or so later, White Hawk and I pulled into the drive of my little bungalow in Red Wing.

It's hard to recall much of the first few days there, except both of us were pretty beat, and there was a lot of cleanup to be done after having left the place to the mercies of the mice and squirrels over the winter.

I remember, after having been there for a week or so, it was time to start thinking about what I could bring for sun dance. I wanted my fourth year's giveaway to be special, so I organized a vehicle-trailer rental from U-Haul. I had a little four-speed Ram pickup I'd bought off the side of the road from a guy who was selling it for the owners, but I couldn't seem to reach the lady listed on the title to have her sign it over to me. White Hawk was trying to help out, kinda; he took over the cooking, ran some errands, even helped out cleaning in the bathroom, but often it seemed he'd help out with the chores he found agreeable, not so much with the other stuff.

I remember he helped a lot when we built a fence and gate across the front of the property at the road. I had what we needed to make it a wheeled double gate, plus the big hinges. It was merely a matter of matching parts to functions, but he began whining, "Why can't we just go to the hardware store and buy what we need?"

"Because we have everything we need here already," I replied and told him I didn't want to argue about it. He helped cut down the sections of fence, but after that was done, he began to put up arguments with almost every proposal I made.

He did know exactly what to do when the little truck's alternator went bad. He installed the replacement from the yard when it was already on the trailer, with only a few days left to spare before purification. He did it in probably one-tenth the time it would have taken me. I have to give him that one. Well done.

However, as Elmer would have said, "Sun dance gettin' really close now." I recall a day when we were getting ready to leave for Rosebud, I'd gathered a large quantity of flat cedar and a well-tanned buffalo robe that I'd bought in Custer, South Dakota, on the way back from the gathering at one of the shopping stops. I had two, so I must have gotten the other one in Rapid City—now that I tot them up, there were several stops, of some several hours' duration each. No wonder the passengers were so antsy; if the situation had been reversed, I'd probably have been even more impatient.

Anyhow, the kitchen supplies from Monkeytown were stored in the garage, and the robes were bagged up in garbage bags, likewise the cedar. I'd gotten a set of artist's acrylic paints somewhere in Wyoming, and I was painting the four buffalo skulls on one of the last days in Minnesota. On one I painted a band of blue above a band of green, for the spotted eagle; one was solid red with a spray of seven yellow circles; one was half-black, half-white with a small red lightning bolt in the middle, for the Heyokas; and the last was a pale sky blue, with a darker four-pointed star in the center, for the morning star (sun dance).

At that time, I'd had no idea it was being called Morningstar Sun Dance. In Santee, it had been the All Nations Sun Dance, then just Ironwood Sun Dance. I just felt something about the morning-star design was right for the fourth skull. The other patterns and colors had to do with Elmer's helping spirits—and the two colors used most with his altar were red and yellow, usually tied as two long cloth streamers at the entrance to his outfit.

Well, there I was painting the skulls, when up into the open driveway comes some young man, soliciting business for some local concern. I can't recall what now. He was obviously very curious about what we were doing, but all I could tell him was that we couldn't be part of what he was selling, as both of us were about to leave for South Dakota the next day. Somehow, his interruption, which brought a brief halt to the work, made the day's events memorable. The pickup was on the trailer, the pin oak tree at the end of the driveway was casting some welcome shade as Hawk wrenched in the new alternator, and the sun shone in a clear sky on a hot Minnesota afternoon.

I'd made it clear to him that under no circumstances were we to bring any *pegi* with us to sun dance. I was having enough guilt going back after seven years—and after having fallen off the wagon—as it was. I began to wish I'd not fallen away, but I know there was no way I could have stayed on then without making things worse. In 2001, after hearing reports about Irene and her bunch smoking reefer in the cookshack, the old man had said, "That *pegi*, we don't want to be nowhere 'round that!"

I was starting to get what are called the sun-dance jitters, and they're not imaginary. I can't recall too much about the trip to Rosebud, even if it took us two days or three. I'd called the kennels to make sure the dogs and cat were all right, and locked up the Red Wing house and latched the gate. We couldn't have made very good time in that high-profile box van pulling that heavy trailer with the Ram on it, but eventually we got there, on the evening of the first of the four days of purification.

I'd had to stop and ask directions again, because Elmer's new location was in a place I'd only been to once before, and the turnoff from the highway came up quickly. Finally, we turned up the long dirt road, past the two hills, and left up to the ridge that gave onto the long downhill lane to his trailer and the sun-dance grounds. As we pulled past the hills, just as we passed the crest of the ridge, it was a little past sundown. There was just enough light to see clearly for a short distance, so it was with a great sense of thankfulness that I saw an eagle fly directly across our path from right to left. It's strange to consider, now, how almost any Native person with even a trace of his or her cultural traditions left will understand why seeing that bird fly in just that way made me feel so good, whereas a non-Native person might just think, *So what?*

CHAPTER 17

Again with the Relatives

WE PULLED IN, AND I WISH I COULD RECALL MORE OF THE events surrounding our arrival, but all I remember is pulling the van off somewhere I could get power, and the Hawk went off with his bedroll to sleep in the ceremony house. The next day was a busy one, as second day always is. The tipis were going up, the fire pit in back of the cookshack (which was the north end of the ceremony house) was being cleaned out and fired up, and the sweat-lodge fires were going morning and evening. I was reacquainting myself with people I hadn't seen in seven years and meeting new ones. I pulled the van around the circular drive in front of Elmer's trailer to unhitch my own trailer with the little Ram on. Then I unloaded the various bundles of things we'd brought, lowered the ramps, drove the Ram off, and took the keys inside to give to the old man. Gilli was around and seemed to be behaving himself, so I told him which bundles were what, and where should I put the buffalo robe? (I'd decided to keep one back for myself.) He pointed out a tipi and said it and the skulls could go in there. I remember being somewhat dismayed by how few people there were, compared to past sun dances.

Now that I recall, it was Hawk who drove the Ram off the trailer, and after my trip to the tipi, I got the keys from him and took them inside with the title to give to the old man. I also had a carton of Camel filters for the old man and a piece of the bear root he used to make the medicine tea he'd have served to us at ceremony. As I said, it was a busy time, and the exact sequence of events is a little hard to recall. Several years later, so much of it is just a blur of sun, dust, and faces.

Elmer hadn't recognized me when I went in back to give him the Ram's keys and title and his smokes. I recall that when I went past Gilli with these gifts, he looked a little put out. I said, "Gilli, I brought some smokes and another piece of that bear root for you." This seemed to mollify him, although his attitude gave me a little worry. What should he expect people to do other than gift the sun-dance chief? It was suspiciously close to jealousy, and I was to learn later on it was even more.

Well, I was pretty anxious about going to see Elmer there in his bedroom, where he was accepting pipes from people who were coming in to pledge, but I did. So anxious I can't recall any of the details of that encounter. Just that I told him I'd brought that pickup as part of my *wopila* for my fourth year, handed him the keys, the title, the cigs, and shook his hand. I came back later to proffer my own pipe, maybe the next day. I recall again being a little shocked to see how frail he'd become—even thinner than he'd been in Santee, if that were possible. He said, *"Hau-hau,"* when I told him of the gifts, then after we shook hands. I left and drove the van and trailer back by the power pole behind the cookshack and hitched the power back up.

The next day, a few more folks showed up, but attendance was still less than half what it had been in Santee. I couldn't help remembering that June and July in Nebraska in 1999, when I'd been there working with him. So many came to be put up on the hill. We took that pickup ride across the county road, past the cattle pasture, back up into the hills where not even his little farmhouse could be seen, after the brief morning sweat. I'd help carry the things, and help with the fire and rocks, but after the fence of ties and flags went up, it was usually four days of wondering how the seeker was doing up there. Then, another trip to pick them up, and they'd return, usually looking pretty weathered, and back into sweat again.

Elmer was always gifted in some way by the seeker, and once in a while Dave Ross or I would receive a little *wopila* for our help. I got a flint and steel fire set once. Later on, in July, this would start to taper off, as folks would start coming into camp for purification. The PA system would be up, and Elmer would tell us what needed to be done. I remember when the Germans arrived—I got along well with them—we went with a few others on a sage-picking run, as instructed. The first year I was there, I'd been fortunate enough to find a sage bud the first time I went picking. The second year, I found another and gifted it to a young lady from Germany. Someone told me it was considered lucky to get one, and I used it to plug my pipe when it was resting in its bag. But in 1999, the Germans and I went up the hill a mile or so north of where the *hanblechiya*, or vision quest, sites were, on the back of a big flatbed trailer pulled by Elmer's old tractor. We'd gathered quite a bit of sages, as the old man would say, and were returning down a pretty steep slope. I was next to one of the German ladies, and as we got going, she started muttering, "*Nein, nein,*" and might have fallen off if I hadn't put an arm around her and held on tight. Later on, she said, "He saved my life." Not really, of course. We always were careful in picking, making sure we didn't pull up roots like he warned us. I'm still thankful I was able to dance with him leading us my first two years; after that, his "poisoned" knee was too painful for him to be out there with us.

IT IS NOW JUNE AGAIN AS I BEGIN REWRITING THIS MEMOIR, AND the angle of the sunlight brings back memories of Santee, when the light's angle was the same that year. Elmer'd been asked to visit at the first day of Steve Red Crow's sun dance, and Patti and I went along.

Patti had been dragging us out to the casino more and more frequently, and at first I enjoyed the novelty, but after my first hour, I didn't like the toxic, overstimulating environment. It was a relief to get away from the old home too and go check out someone else's sun dance. The grounds were on a flat tableland out behind the house, where we'd been for the funeral some months earlier. As we drove in, a shirtless young man wearing a bone choker pulled out the coffee can with the cedar chips in it and smudged us off. The dancers were resting, and one Indian man was carrying the eagle staff out to rest against the sun dance tree, but he was called back and left it standing in the earth. I can't recall Elmer's remarks to the dancers, but what did leave an impression was how one of the white dancers who was still out in the dance circle went up to the eagle staff and just held it lightly, without moving it from its position. He got called on it by someone and relinquished it immediately, but Patti took it in the worst way, as evidence that the white dancers were "trying to steal our ceremonies." She even brought up her opinion over the microphone during the evening address to the sun dancers at that year's dance. Perhaps I'm wrong, but I didn't see it like that. He may have been overeager to pick it up, but it seemed like Patti was trying to squeeze as much mileage out of it as she could.

Earlier in the summer, one afternoon when Elmer, Pete, and I were resting from our labors, she got to talking about some local land dispute between the tribe and a local rancher, something to do with leases for grazing cattle, and her point was that to most of the white folks around there, an Indian wasn't worth as much to them as a cow. Her son, Jamie, was also present and recalled an incident from when he'd been employed in construction on the then-new Chief Standing Bear Memorial Bridge. One of his coworkers had delivered that old Western racist chestnut right to his face: "The only good Indian is a dead Indian." This was the same bridge we'd used to cross over to South Dakota to visit Red Crow's family and to get to sun dance.

To jump forward one year, it was also in early June that I'd gone to Patti's ceremony. She'd wrapped the stem of her *canunpa* up in prayer ties and announced that the spirits had told her she was to run her own monthly ceremony. It was after this she'd talked me into putting my original sun-dance *canunpa* up on the hill.

When I did go in to *opagi* Elmer, not too much was said. He had me sign the notebook, with my address and contact info first, then we got down to it. I recall him puffing away, sitting on his narrow bed. He was starting to get a little cranky and short-tempered; at the Rainbow Gathering, I'd made the mistake of neglecting to remove my hearing aid before I'd gone in for a bath in the creek—which washed it right out of my head. There was no time for a replacement in Red Wing, so when he began to speak after the pipe was out and he'd handed it back to me, I had to say, "What?"

He exclaimed, "Goddamn it, you listen!"

I explained in a rush, "Elmer, I am listening. I just lost my hearing aid, and I'm going deaf." A little exaggeration, maybe, but it mollified him.

He backed off a bit, let his head down, and said, "I been sick—so sick I can't walk."

That was as close as he'd ever come to saying sorry. I don't recall much more of this exchange, but once my info was in the book and this bit of repartee was over, I got out of there.

There were a number of his kids there besides Gilli, and their children and relations, and they were taking advantage of the old man's infirmity, as well as being a probable cause of it. White Hawk, at one point after he'd gone in to meet Elmer, came back out and told me there were a couple of young'uns sitting on the living room couch, smoking pot. Even he was shocked by this. Well, I told a couple of the senior sun dancers, and we put a stop to that.

I recall the previous day, after I'd unloaded all the gifts with the Hawk's help, that I'd gotten reacquainted with Nico from Santee and Don, a Native guy I'd first met at Santee sun dance back in 1997 or 1998. He'd admired the double-hitch knot I'd tied to get my tent up, and we'd gotten to talking. We both got huge grins on when we saw each other, and with Nico as a third, we proceeded to catch up on seven years' worth of history. I told them how I'd come to leave Elmer's in 2001, the sunstroke, and being fed up with Gilli, and they likewise filled me in. Later on that first day, when things finally cooled off for the evening, I saw Don take the old man out and around the sun-dance grounds on a tour of inspection. It was then I realized I'd made a mistake in getting a vehicle with a clutch for the old man. The right knee, the one that had been witched by a jealous powwow dancer so many years before, made it impossible for him to drive the thing himself. But that worked out, for he was soon to have a driver who would be that and more, and would be with him up until the end of his life.

CHAPTER 18

Gwen and Sage

THIS WAS A YOUNG SINGLE MOTHER, GWEN, AND HER NINE-year-old boy, Sage, who were newcomers to Elmer's sun dance that year. Homeless, victims of a house fire caused by a leaky gas line, Gwen had offered her boy a choice between staying on where they were and starting over there or going to see his relatives on the Rosebud rez. One of Crow Dog's sons was Sage's father, and they'd been planning on attending his sun dance, held just a few miles away, but had been unceremoniously evicted by a couple who told them they were in "their" camping spot. They got run off, so they came over to Elmer's. Gwen was originally from California, somewhere in the Inland Empire region, but had been living in Rapid City and serving the Lakota people in Pine Ridge for some sixteen years. Sage was as well-mannered and likeable a young man as any nine-year-old could be. Cheerful and helpful, not given to whining, he put the manners of most other kids his age I've met to shame.

Also present were some of Elmer's sons I'd never met before and some of his daughters and grown grandkids. The big campground south of the cookshack was filling up now, and by the end of the second day, the work of getting the pine boughs into place on the arbor and around the perimeter of the dance circle was well under way.

Jason and Konda had shown up, a couple from Lincoln who'd been coming to the old man's ceremonies and sun dances since his early years in Santee, maybe even before that at Ironwood. I can still hear his shrill, reedy tenor pealing across the prairie at 4:00 a.m.: "*Hoka hey*, sun dancers! The grandfathers are waiting," referring to the stones being heated to red-hot in the fires he'd lit and had been tending for some two hours. Had to have, since having done the same thing myself so many times for ceremony in Santee, I know how long it takes to cook 'em.

The Germans had also arrived, Ulee and his wife and the others. Ulee's wife had the bad luck to begin her moon time just after getting off the plane. She was set up in a little tent by herself, just on the other side of the barbed-wire fence, a little ways south of the gate. A woman in that condition can't be involved or even present at any ceremony. You may call it primitive sexism, but I've heard too many stories about medicine men getting really sick when this taboo was violated.

Gwen, Gorgie, Lorna, and the other ladies were keeping busy at the cookshack, feeding the dancers, supporters, and relatives until it was time for the dancers to fast. They also kept track of the food gifts brought by so many and made sure none of it wandered off, so the surplus would be at Elmer's disposal, which is how it's supposed to be. Also present was a young lady I'd never seen before, called Nancy. This would-be helper was a problem. Content with her task as dishwasher and cookware wrangler, she was loud, prissy, controlling, and unreasonable. When sometime during the second day Elmer's big, black shepherd mix, Hokshila, was penned up with Sage's puppy Hampa (Fatty) so as to be kept away from the dance, Nancy objected to my borrowing a pan to get them some water; there was no shade where they were. She even mouthed off to me, saying, "You don't need to worry about them. They're sun-dance dogs. They're tough." Which made no frickin' sense, then or now. I refused to start an argument with anyone during purification, but those dogs got their water.

By this time, I'd gotten my ties and flags made and had set myself up as the smudger at the gate. It was something that had been done faithfully at all three sun dances I'd attended in Santee. I smudged off every incoming vehicle with cedar and tied a strip of colored cloth to the antenna, in token of correct entry. I had a little shade arbor and tipi to myself, and Allen, one of the old-timers who'd been an Eagle dancer since Santee at least, came over and told me that this hadn't been done at Elmer's sun dances for years. We got to talking about Elmer, how he'd said the spirits were going to give him one more year, but Allen said Elmer wanted to die. When I asked him how he knew, he said, "He told me."

By the third day of purification, most of the work on the arbor and cookshack was done, and White Hawk left with Gwen to do a little work for her on a homesite she'd been given per-mission to build on. He came back angry and told me she'd lost it and yelled at him. The details were sketchy, and are all gone now, but at the time, I took his part. I didn't like Gwen at first. She was loud and would complain if anything happened that she didn't like. I thought Sage was a great kid, but his mom was so direct as to verge on bad manners. Since then, I've reversed that opinion; White Hawk turned out to be a lousy worker—for me, at least—and Gwen and I are close friends.

Later on, I had occasion to leave my post at the gate and go on a sage-gathering run with some folks. When I got back, the Hawk came up to me excitedly and said, "Oh, man, you missed it. Some of the senior women took Nancy up the hill over there, past the dance circle, and laid into her for mouthing off to a sun dancer. They went back and saged off the spot later, it was so intense." I saw Nancy a little while after that, and she looked chastened, to say the least; one could see she'd been crying. Ordinarily, I'd feel some sympathy for someone in her situation, but not this time. She'd brought it all on herself and in a way had been fortunate; at some sun dances, she would've been told to leave.

I think it was later that afternoon that my opinion of Gwen began to change. She and Sage were sitting in the shade between my tall van and Elmer's old school bus, where he kept all the sun-dance and ceremonial paraphernalia. It didn't run, but it had a lock that bore the marks of several attempted break-ins. She was talking to another lady, and gazing at them, I felt this strong sense of connection, or at least of significance.

It is difficult now, even at such a short remove as five to six years, to distinguish events of the 2008 sun dance from the one that followed; so many events were similar. But I recall being introduced to some of the newcomers at Elmer's circle as a sun dancer and former fire keeper. And early in the afternoon of the third day, the last of the ceremonial tipis belonging to Elmer was to be put up, and my assistance was requested. Fortunately, having been shown the right way to do this in Santee, and having done it several times, I found it's kinda like riding a bicycle— once you've learned ...

So there I was, after looping the top of the tripod and placing them to the west, north, and south, directing the newbies in the placement of the poles, while I served as rope man and walked that rope around and around. The rope must be some forty feet long to accommodate the height and additional poles and then tie the cover on and tie off the end below. Before this, the completed frame is expanded or contracted to fit the cover, and the door-way is always to the east. One always walks the rope and places the poles in a sunwise manner. When all but the last two longest, slenderest poles are left, the canvas cover is tied on, let fall, and pulled around the frame. The last two poles are for the "ears," the smoke flaps above the opening, and are adjustable.

I remember, at the last sun dance in Santee, Elmer was still in teasing mode after my stunt in picking up the hundred-pound propane tank. After I'd helped with the poles on that one, he picked up the heavy bundle of canvas and said, "Hey, muscleman!" and just pointed with a jerk of his chin up at the top. He was jokingly challenging me to climb up there, when this job's always left to a small boy. Everyone had a good laugh, and I had to beg off.

"Elmer, I couldn't do it, I'm too fat and heavy." Which was mostly true then and is really true now.

I remember telling the young man who'd asked me to help put up the tipi and who was directing the final touches on the grounds, "It's been about ten years since I've done this."

Dino, a middle-aged Ponca fellow from the Santee days, one of the leaders, and Gilli were basically leading us in the dance that year, since Elmer was too ill to lead us himself, let alone come out and dance. The fourth day of purification was tree day, and sometime around the middle of the afternoon, most of the camp set out to bring in the grandfather, as the tree is called once it's cut. It was down along a gravel road at the bottom of the hill from Elmer's, a good distance, some two or three miles, and just past Crow Dog's Paradise. A little creek ran along the other side of the road, and it was much cooler and shadier than up on the table-land where the grounds and Elmer's trailer were.

I recall that the young boy and girl who took the first swings with the ax barely chipped the bark, and then the older ones took over. I took a turn or two, along with most of the rest of the men, and soon the beautiful cottonwood, with twin forks high and low, was ready to fall. This was the crucial moment. A score or so of us had long ash stringers from the arbor, and we lined up two men to a limb along the path where it looked to fall. No matter how heavy it is, the grandfather must not be allowed to touch the ground. If a few of the leaves and branches of the highest parts do so, that's not important; it's the main trunk and the forks that count. This was a tall one, and it was a job to catch it. Once the final few cuts were taken with the axe, and the trunk began to sway, we all raised our stringers high and took the weight. The next thing was to carry it over and set it on a long flatbed trailer. It had to go butt first, and much care was taken not to let anyone step on or over any of the trailing branches. Warnings and calls of "Look out!" were constantly being shouted. It was set in place and tied down, and I called to Dino, "Dino! Do you want me to lash the crown?"

He called back, "Yes!"

So I took a long, red nylon rope and carefully wound it around the upper limbs of the tree, drawing the upper branches above the main fork up and inward. Then I tied it off, and we were good to go.

Since the putting up of the tree, the tying of the ceremonial objects in the fork, the tying-on of the pledgers' ropes and flags, and the winding of the hundreds of prayer ties around the base of the trunk are the next steps in the ceremony, I'm not going to describe any of these in detail. More information can be found in the works of Native authors who have the authority and under-standing to speak of these things. I can only say that I was afraid of a repeat of the sunstroke, which would again prevent me from finishing fourth year. But apparently the grandfathers judged my heart was good for this dance, because a curious thing happened.

Far from getting stroked out, my skin, which I'd not tanned and toughened through exposure, never once even burned through the four days of dancing. It kept getting redder and red-der and more painful with each passing day, until even the small spots of direct sunlight that found their way through the pine-bough walls of the rest arbor felt like bee stings. But I just took that pain and prayed even harder with it as you're supposed to do—just focus on that tree and pray.

I was dancing that year for Leonard Peltier, the falsely accused, wrongly convicted, and FBI-railroaded AIM member who is serving two consecutive life sentences for two killings everyone, even the FBI, knows he didn't commit. Another one of their many COINTELPRO scapegoats/victims. His final parole hearing was happening at the same time as the dance, and I told as many people as I could to pray for his release. But he remains in prison, the further victim of unprovoked, murderous prison attacks no doubt authored by our shadow rulers in cahoots with federal prison personnel. Don't tell me that America is a democracy, the land of the free. You're only free in this country if you're a rich, white, Anglo-Saxon male. Everybody else lives under a different, much harsher law that is altered to fit the situation at the discretion of the police state.

Instead of catching up, I seem to have gotten ahead of myself. Back on the evening of the second day, Gwen and I were out past the cookshack, nearly to the lower gate. We'd taken out some trash to the big Dumpster, at least she had, and I'd been out by my van. I had some solar panels mounted on top of the heavy vinyl roof, leading directly to four deep-cycle batteries on a shelf formed by the van's interior that were connected to an inverter. White Hawk had been doing some rewiring for me, putting in fusible links and generally improving the setup. Unfortunately, he was one of those kinds of workers who are apt to leave a job in the middle, with tools and parts left lying around, and stray off onto something else. I was beginning to wish I'd left him in Wyoming; nothing steams me more than to have to be picking up after someone who's supposed to be helping me. His work was OK, but the execution was sloppy.

I'd just gotten done straightening up after his latest space-out and was in kind of a foul mood when Gwen came up just as I caught sight of something that froze my blood. There, perched on the power pole just inside the fence, was a huge owl, staring at us. It looked to be a great horned, although in the dark, lit only by the eerie green glow of the sodium-vapor safety lamp, it was hard to tell. We both saw it at the same time. Gwen asked, "Karl, is that an owl?"

"Yup, sure is," I replied.

Again, this may be something that most non-Native readers won't understand, while most Native readers will understand immediately why I found it so chilling. I think I've already mentioned my own bad experiences with them, but to enlarge, most tribes regard the owl as a messenger of sickness, death, and disaster. None of them with any sense will have anything to do with their feathers. I felt a gloom cast on my expectations for this sun dance. This was a bad omen, just about the worst. I found out later that a male relative of Elmer's, an older man with a seemingly perpetually angry demeanor, had promised rewards to the kids if they'd hurl stones at the bird and drive it off. I think it flew off for a bit, after Gwen and I started talking about it, but it came back. Worst of all, one of the kids did hit it and knocked loose a feather that White Hawk found the next day and kept with him. He told me later on of his betrayal by his family, his rage and desire for vengeance, and of how an owl had come and promised to help him. He believed this and referred to his owl medicine. While I'm not sure if White Hawk ever did get his revenge, the owls coming to Elmer's did turn out to be a significant omen—I heard later on that there were several deaths in the Running family that summer and fall.

The Hawk came and told me all this—the stone-throwing and his affinity—with the feather he'd found in his hand. Told me he'd found it right under where the bird had been perched. I told him I didn't like having it around, but I agreed to let him store it in the van while he went off to do that little bit of work for Gwen, which ended badly. I'd cleaned up his mess and restored his most recent rewiring of my solar setup to where it had been before his latest tinkering, leaving in the fuses.

Purification is for letting go of negative thoughts, the concerns of the white world, and focusing on one's prayers. There is, however, always a challenge, embedded in the fabric of this world and concerning that ceremony in particular, it seems. This time, it was having him and that feather around me. We'd had some words on the trip up about our respective buddies, when he'd called some crows flying by "ugly birds." That got my back up, since they've always helped me out since I began trying to walk the red road. I told him not to talk like that and learned about his past and his owl medicine. What he had told me seemed like genuine assistance, but from the dark side of the spirit world, since the main motivation was anger, and the goal seemed to be vengeance. That should have told me we'd never agree, since crows and owls are mortal enemies, but I thought it could be worked around.

He'd come back from his attempt to help Gwen fairly disgruntled, telling me that Gwen had lost it and screamed at him. He wasn't too clear on the details, but it sounded pretty unfair. From then on, I sort of took the attitude that I wouldn't have anything more to do with her. If only I'd known I was backing a lame horse.

Hawk had filled in for me a few times on smudging incoming vehicles at the main gate and had reported that some carloads of Indians had seemed downright hostile about it. Neither of us could suss out if it was because it was being done at all or because it was a couple of *wasicus* doing it, although the Hawk could pass for half. The worst part was the deal with the Indian kids and the hatchet. I had a nice one I used for chopping the cedar and firewood, and one or the other of them stole it. There were three little boys and a couple *wincincalas*, and I'd trusted them to chop a little wood for me since they seemed to want something to do. I'd left the gate for a little while, and when I came back, the hatchet was gone.

When I asked them sharply where it was, one of the older boys said they hadn't been there the whole time, but, he said, "thought I saw somebody walking away over there." For a half second, I almost believed him. But of course they'd stolen it. Reminded me of the generator fiasco back in Santee. After I'd resolved that by buying Elmer and Patti a new one, Grandpa mentioned something like, "Some of them Indians, they like to steal." That was one of the worst things about Rosebud: You came in, desiring to be of some service to the people, and you get ripped off for your trouble. Ordinarily, I'd take it as a teaching on nonattachment, but it's worse somehow when little kids are doing it. And when the people are so sunk in feeding their habits and thirst for alcohol that they literally steal the sacred things from one of their own holy men, that's the worst too. It just drags you down. You lose faith. I saw quite clearly why Elmer had left his tribe so many years before and gone to practice his calling among the Isanti Nakota of Nebraska, even on land that had originally been ceded to the Ponca. His own kin just did him in.

When I told Jason about the theft later on, he just said, "If all you got taken for was a hatchet, you got off easy."

The sun dance of 2008 was the first time I'd attempted to fast all four days. I did all right, too, except that the morning of the second day, I attempted to sustain my energies with a swig or two from a carton of whole milk I had on hand. Not solid food, and not water, and even fasting dancers are permitted to take a little broth, or some such. This was when I found out for a definite fact that I'm lactose intolerant. My stomach clenched up like a fist, and a nasty queasy feeling came over me. Nonetheless, I managed to complete that day's dancing.

I've already described how kind the sun was to me, how even after not "toughening up" my skin, I never burned, even after all four days. By the end of the second day, though, I was really dragging. I had to put something on my abused stomach to help it get over the last of the milk. So I had a little cooked cornmeal in a small plastic pouch. The whole of it barely covered the palm of my hand. I ate that that evening, with a prayer that I be excused, because Elmer had said that things needed to be done in the old way as the old-time sun dancers had done them. No eating and absolutely no water for the dancers, which had always been the rule, anyway. I confess to inadvertently breaking that one; the exact wording I had was that the dancers were not to touch water. We were allowed coffee in the morning, since it was not exactly water and certainly not food, but when I went to add a little creamer to it, there in my camper, the condensation from the bottle made contact. I see now, I could simply have grabbed it with a towel or something, but since I didn't drink any, I had a feeling it wasn't really an issue.

The point of that dance is to suffer and to offer one's suffering to those above—so that the people may live, so that all life may continue. What with my tenderized hide, sour stomach, and increasing exhaustion, by the end of the third day, I had plenty to offer! I recall that I was looking rough enough by the end of the dance round that one of the senior leaders sorta ran over to me and fanned me down with his eagle wing, muttering some reproachful comments on the state of my intelligence. The fanning helped, and I wish I could remember who it was and what was said. White Hawk told me later that instead of stepping to each of the drumbeats, I was managing about one in four. But I remember that as a good day. I was praying hard for Leonard, trying not to think of myself, and offering my suffering to the grandfather tree.

Apart from my own experience, the only thing I will say about that dance is that I'm glad it was Dino, rather than Gilli, who pierced me. I had pledged myself to drag buffalo skulls that year, in atonement for falling off the wagon and getting one of my little dogs run over thereby. This had happened in 2005, within a few weeks of my buying the first bottle of wine. I had thought, since Patti talked me into putting my *canunpa* up on the hill in Santee after her bogus ceremony, that the connection with Elmer's altar, and the spirits, was broken. But the words of the old man had come back to me: "If somebody picks up that pipe, then puts it down, they don't go much farther." This had worried me, but as I later found out, that and other things had come back on Patti. The connection was there, had always been there, and now I was wanted, as I realized when they came into my little upstairs room and pounded on the wall once I'd gotten another pipe.

So, I was wrong. The connection was there all along, and my poor little shih tzu had to pay the price. I won't go into details, but an owl had flown across the route I was driving on the day she was killed. That let me know the spirits had arranged it. I don't blame them; they had to do it. After all, I'd been warned; an elder from Isanti had come to address the dancers and supporters in 1999. He'd said, "Drinking and drugs and this *canunpa* don't mix." It was my fault.

But getting back, Dino had pierced me so lightly that once the pegs were in my back and I started walking, I broke free before I'd taken four steps. As White Hawk told me later, "The skulls just popped up once, and then you broke."

I heard Gilli ask Dino why he'd gone in so shallow, and he'd said, "I don't want to hurt anybody."

To which Gilli replied, "If I'd pierced him, he woulda drug skulls."

I also seem to recall that Gwen had made the tremolo call, what they call the "brave heart" sound, when I was out there. That's a sign of honor, and I'm grateful to her for it, but I don't feel I deserved it.

One more thing from purification: Elmer's younger brother, Al Running, had come up to me and complimented me on the bear-claw necklace I was wearing. It was a single claw, suspended on a braided white leather thong. I'd traded for it at the Rainbow Gathering, and I told him it wasn't a claw at all but a carved piece of fossil mammoth ivory. He seemed happy to hear it, and I think he was being so polite because I'd brought up the Dodge Ram and gifts for the sun dance for his brother.

There's not too much more to tell of the 2008 sun dance, except that after the four days of fasting, the feasting afterward was especially welcome. We received the usual admonishments from Grandpa about resting for four days afterward, and indeed, I wasn't quite ready to go back out into the world just yet. After the intensity of the all-day dance, plus the fasting, one is left in an altered state. As Elmer said back in 1999, "Least we could stay outta them casinos." Nonetheless, I managed a short trip out from Elmer's outfit during this time. I was trying to keep the trips short. I took just a quick run to Mission, the largest town on the rez, at first. While I was there at the store getting supplies, I got cornered on the way in by an older Lakota woman, who begged me for some money, saying, "I didn't eat for three days." I was tempted to snap back with, "I got that beat," but thought better of it and handed her all my pocket change, and she thanked me, saying, "I'll tell all those snakes and turtles not to bite you, when you go in swimmin'." OK. Then we headed back.

On the next day, Nico, the Hawk, and I were going to some entertainment, or maybe it was the annual Rosebud Powwow, and we wanted Jason, the fire tender, to come along with us. He was wary of leaving, saying he feared the relatives would vandalize his vehicle if he left. It was around this time that I tried to get him to fill me in on some of the events of the past seven years, especially the time when I'd house-sat for Elmer in the late winter of 2001. He was going on the road then to do ceremony for some folks, and when he left, he told me, "In the mornin', take a little spoon of coffee and pour it out, and say, 'That's for Elmer Runnin'.'"

My stint was uneventful, but during another trip, one of his married sons, at the instigation of his crazy, diabetic wife, had gone through the old man's trailer and cleaned him out, leaving the place a shambles. I know this since it happened before the 2001 sun dance and because I'd talked to the lady in question just before monthly ceremony late the previous fall. She was at the hospital and called to get a ride. When no one was willing to miss ceremony on her account, I'd hung up, but she'd called back, very angry, and threatened a nonspecific vengeance. Also, the trailer was parked at Norman and Shannon's by the time I got back, and he told me they'd done it. I wanted to know how things had gone for the old man when he was over there, but Jason wouldn't tell me. "You don't want to know," was all he'd say.

I'd also met a (more or less) recent arrival at Elmer's altar, a Southern fellow called Lehr. Turned out that Lehr had spent some time with the old man during my absence, helping and learning, and had been so incensed with Norman's treatment of Elmer that he wanted to shoot him. But Elmer had said, "Don't shoot Norman; he's my boy."

I'd met Lehr during a spring monthly ceremony in 2001, and he'd gone into sweat shortly after having eaten a tuna sandwich. When he'd come out, he'd complained of the difficulty he'd had with a full stomach in there. "Don't ever go into sweat with a full stomach," I told him. It seems as though Lehr, for a time at least, had come to fill in the gap in support the old man needed, left by my own absence.

Getting back to the day of rest, however, we waited by the little market in Mission for Jason for nearly twenty minutes, after having arranged to meet him there, but we left after that, thinking he wasn't going to show. He did, eventually.

The second day after the dance, I was still pretty out of it. It was becoming clearer why the sun dance had originally been a twelve-day ceremony. Even without having undergone the fantastic rigors experienced by the old-timers, one still needed some little while to adjust to "normality" again.

As our interpreter, after every dance in Santee, Elmer had made a speech to us over the PA. Many of his speeches had to do with how the dancers were to conduct themselves, admonishing us to "stay quiet, to talk straight, always. Don't talk behind." And especially not to go around to different sun dances. Once the pine boughs were off the arbors, however, and taken down to Crow Dog's, it was hard to sit around camp doing nothing. So I went off with Nico and the Hawk once again, this time to the town of Saint Francis to the Rosebud Museum there. I was hoping to find an English-Lakota dictionary in the gift shop.

We headed over there, and lo and behold, the museum was open, and they had the dictionary. However, as we pulled up, we noticed a bit of a confrontation nearby. A Lakota man had just exited a parked vehicle and had exchanged some sharp words with whoever was inside and then slammed the car door angrily. I started over to a convenience store across the street, not realizing this guy was trailing me. He'd just gotten up behind me when the Hawk caught up with him and sorta deflected him. No doubt he would have been, at the least, an insistent panhandler. I found the groceries we were looking for at the store, plus a black-and-yellow beadwork spider I liked. Shoulda listened to Grandpa and stayed in camp.

On the third day, I started on my flags and ties for *wopila*, the giving of thanks to the spirits for the sun dance and for prayers granted. The campground was mostly empty, only one or two tents left. At her invitation, I sat in Lorna's tipi as I worked. She was one of the senior lady dancers and had been with the old man since at least the years in Santee.

I'd done a bit of scavenging on the campground and found several braids of sweet grass, a new-looking stock tub, and a deep purple blanket, which I'd claimed.

Gwen and Sage were staying on, too, as it turned out. Sometime during the dance, Elmer had come up to Gwen and said, "The spirits, what they told me, you should stay here and take care of me." She'd agreed, and as things turned out, the spirits never did a better day's work than that. Unfortunately, the appointment, as it were, of a rank newcomer to such a close position to the *wicasa wakan* caused some jealousy among those who should have known better, or at least had more respect.

Gwen and Sage had begun to move into the trailer and were making themselves at home. Gwen began to take on her role as Elmer's cook and caretaker. Some of the relatives—namely, Gilli and a grandson named Anthony Running, known as Iktomi, and his woman—were staying on for a while. Sage had an adorable shepherd–rez dog mix puppy called Hampa, or "Fatty." It was a good fit, as Sage and Hampa were both good-natured and agreeable.

As to the Hawk and myself, the four days were almost over, and it was time to think about heading home. One of the things Elmer had told us, in his customary harangues during purification, was: "The spirits, what they told me, if we do things right, they're gonna give me one more year."

I was worried about having *technically* touched water and the half handful of corn I'd eaten, but directly after the dance, during the feasting, we saw some eagles flying overhead toward the east. I was still mostly deaf from the loss of the hearing aid, but a young Lakota lady remarked in my hearing that one of them was rattling as it flew. This we all took as a good sign, as we took the grandfather tree out the east gate, that things had gone well. I asked her what kind of rattle it sounded like—a deer hoof, or a turtle shell? "More like a deer hoof," she told me. Wish I could have heard that.

I had brought a bunch of possessions from Red Wing, in addition to the Ram and the dance paraphernalia, and I used these as my fourth-year *wopila*, or giveaway. There was always a giveaway after the dance; either someone was finishing a fourth year or giving thanks for prayers answered. I had a few choice items, and Lehr also had some nice things out. Nico got a copy of a Stratocaster guitar from me, and I got a huge hand-carved wooden spoon from Lehr. Nico told me he was going to be around a lot, after that, swinging by to help look after the old man, work on vehicles as needed, and so on. Soon afterward, I learned that Peltier's final chance at parole had been denied, undoubtedly due to pressure from the fascist thugs of the FBI swaying the parole board's decision. Nico's promises were to prove equally empty.

However, Nico did me one more service that year. We had taken a trip out to the rez dump, just to prospect, the last of the four days, and I'd mentioned to him that I wanted to get a special tattoo to commemorate finishing my fourth year. He said that he knew of a local artist, a Rosebud guy. We struck out at the dump and then went and found the artist at home. After I'd had him sketch out the designs I had in mind, Nico drove me out to the nearest ATM, and I withdrew the necessary cash.

But back in Lorna's tipi, I was having a little much-needed quiet time, working on the flags and ties for *wopila*. My mind would wander a bit, flashing back to the dance and even further back to Santee. One morning there, I'd taken a coffee break about midmorning, while Elmer had kept on working. This was about the time we were cleaning up the parking area after the heavy rains. I'd mentioned to Patti that he was pretty energetic for a man pushing eighty, and she'd said that he'd once told her, "My work's the only thing keeps me going."

I need to mention that Lorna had been very helpful earlier. I'd gotten a signed-over title to the Dodge Ram before I'd taken it home to Red Wing. I'd been impressed by the fact that it had started right up after having sat by the side of the road for nearly a year. I ended up paying half again as much in repairs to get it past inspection in Minnesota, but unfortunately there was a co-owner's name on the title that hadn't been signed off on. I'd tried getting in touch with the female individual before we'd left for sun dance, but I'd had no luck. In order for Elmer to get the title and registration in his name, that signature had to be there, and when I'd explained to Lorna that the vehicle was all paid for and fixed up and that nothing truly underhanded was involved, she'd agreed to sorta fill in the blank.

So I was grateful to her for that and glad to be sitting in her tipi, when who should come up but Nico and his girlfriend. I'd meant to spend at least one of the four days in camp, as I'd oughta, but Nico came with a pack of my brand of cigarettes, American Spirit Lights, and a requested a favor. When someone brings you tobacco, that's a sign of respect, and if you take it, you're more or less obligated to honor the request. He and his lady needed some help getting her the proper uniforms for the new medical facility job she was about to start, and they were skint. Nico also needed some work gear, so it was necessary to put the flags and ties aside and head on down the road to Valentine, Nebraska.

We had fun, despite the fact that I was still somewhat punchy. I recall we stopped at a church that was having a basement flea market, and we all found some stuff. I had hit an ATM and gotten them the wherewithal for the uniforms, and at the sale I found a heavy plastic flare gun, still in its case with several flares. On the way home, Nico's lady asked me why I needed such a thing.

"Don'tcha remember that one episode of *Johnny Quest?*" I answered quickly. "Where Race Bannon uses a flare gun to set fire to the deck of the bad guys' speedboat after puncturing their gas tank? Huh? Don'tcha?"

She just rolled her eyes and muttered, "Only a guy."

Since then, that 1960s animated kids' show has been rebroad-
cast several times, and I've taken up watching it. Turns out, I was
manufacturing that sequence of events from whole cloth; there's
no such episode. But I digress. Told ya I was still punchy.

To return to the previous night, Nico had dropped me off at
a housing development somewhere near Soldier Creek, where the
tattoo artist lived. After knocking, I went into the little house,
one of a number of BIA units, where the artist—who traded
under the name HostileInk—did his thing. I laid out the cash
we'd agreed on, and he began setting up his gear. The first thing
was to clear up some details of the designs.

When I'd been sitting in my little shade arbor during purification, doing security, I'd looked up suddenly one afternoon,
feeling my attention being drawn out of myself. Two good-looking horses had just come around to the near side of one of the
innumerable prairie hills, about a mile off, and were looking at
me intently. There are more than a few Indian families with the
surname Looking Horse or Horses Looking, and it seemed I knew
why just in that moment. There was some significance about it I
can't explain. So one tattoo was to be of the hills, the horses, and
the eagle that had flown across our path the night we'd arrived.
That was the left wrist. The right one was four spiders inside four
four-pointed stars in the four colors. The artist used a "ledger
art" style.

The placement of the tattoos was for the same reason a lot
of the old-timers, Elmer included, had their wrists tattooed.
According to Lakota belief, after a person dies and begins his
or her journey to the other side, he or she has to cross a ridge
guarded by an Owl Woman. If your wrists are tattooed, she lets
you go on. If not, she throws you back, and you become a *wanagi*, or ghost. As was said to me by one of the Indian dancers, I
think just after the dance, when I was obviously feeling down,
"Hey, Karl, this life's pretty simple. First we're on this side,

then we go over to that side." More telepathy, or so I suspect; they were gently spoken words of comfort. I'd been in a bit of a turmoil: Elmer hadn't remembered me from Santee; Grandma Darlene was visiting from Minneapolis, was nearly bedridden herself, and was treating Gwen (and anyone else who'd go along with it) like a servant, insisting on being babysat; and I'd found I couldn't depend on the Hawk to finish anything he started. But despite it all, I managed to finish my fourth year, I'd gotten a tattoo after every one of my previous dances, and these were to be the last.

HostileInk's house had other occupants and guests, some four or five young men, and as they entered through the kitchen door (carrying a case of beer), the artist cautioned them not to walk too closely behind him for fear of upsetting his inks and needle gun, or whatever it's called. They were loud and boisterous, but not crazy. They offered me a beer, but I declined. I'd had enough of that kind of fun. They also started smoking *pegi* and offered me some of that too, but I had to say no again. I was returning to Elmer's camp and didn't wish to be disrespectful. All this must have been taking place on the evening of the third day. I recall the artist giving me some gel to help with the healing process. He also warned me not to get them wet, or the ink would bleed out and they would fade more quickly. I mention this because I distinctly remember having a bath in Elmer's tub the next day, and having to wrap my bandaged wrists in plastic secured by rubber bands to keep them dry.

I recall that the Hawk and I spent a day or two after the last of the four rest days, helping Gwen and Jason and Konda clean up the house and grounds and secure the donated food items. Almost no one else had stayed very long after the dance. As soon as the feasting and giveaways on the last day were over, there was a whole line of vehicles making their way up the long lane to the cattle gate at the top of the ridge. A lot of gear plus the usual extra food supplies had been left on the grounds, and there was a lot of work to be done. The relatives began to absent themselves. Gilli wasn't around much, or Norman, or Webster.

I forgot to mention one incident during purification. A party from Alabama had set up their camp on the southeast corner of the camping area. On the second day, Elmer got on the PA and said that the spirits had told him that some in camp were smoking *pegi* and talking on their cell phones. Once you were in for purification, communication with the outside world wasn't supposed to take place; pot smoking certainly wasn't. On the afternoon of the third day, a little bit of a windstorm got up. I say a little bit; compared to the twisters that region produces, it was minor. The tipis stayed up, most of the camp was intact, but every tent of the Alabamians was flattened. They left the next morning, and at least they'd picked up, but their wreckage nearly filled the big Dumpster outside the main gate. Turns out they were the cell-phone talkers, the ones that got it. It reminded me of the flood in Santee. How the spirits had done their own bit in purifying the grounds.

The weather had been very good for the dance, but the wind picked up again afterward. I recall having to chase down a lot of plastic bags and whatnot that had blown into the barbed-wire fence. A white rancher lived not far off—he ran cattle on the land he leased from Elmer. We had to call Lala, Elmer's big, black shepherd mix back from running them, now that the dogs were free. Lala had only three legs, the left hind one having been shot off by this same rancher, when he'd caught him at it before. The man was also a drunk.

The day we left dawned windless and clear. I spent the morning helping Gwen load the last of the leftover groceries into the freezer in the cookshack and hauling bag after bag of trash out to the Dumpster. By the time we were done, there was almost the same volume as the Dumpster's contents piled up outside it. I was anxious to be off, because the previous afternoon, I'd gotten a sudden worrying concern about my boarded dogs. Just a sudden premonition that I needed to be back with them.

As it turned out, I was right. One of my little shih tzus had developed an eye infection due to being neither groomed nor bathed during the nearly two months of my absence. This was contrary to my instructions to the people whom I thought I could trust. They ran a little private, no-kill shelter in Papillion, Nebraska. The kennel paid for the surgery, since the infection had abscessed and the eye ruptured, but I never boarded any of my critters there again. The Hawk and I could not return to Minnesota immediately, not until she was well enough to travel, but eventually, by summer's end, I caught up with him there, having given him the keys to the place and sent him on ahead sometime in September.

I have to skip over all the ups and downs I had with White Hawk; they're not germane to this book. The very short of it was that he found a girlfriend, and I had to change the plan, which was to let him overwinter one year as a caretaker. I'd been feeding him all summer and paying him for more work per week than he admitted he'd been doing—but I was seeing less and less in return and getting more argument for my trouble. At least I waited until he had somewhere to go before I gave him the sack. I've often wished we'd parted on better terms, but when I was cleaning out the closet I'd lent him for his own, I found that owl's feather lying on the floor under a pile of his things—this, after he told me he'd gotten rid of it. Afterward, when he'd driven up in his girlfriend's car, claimed his stuff, and left, I saw a big owl lift up out of the woods across the road and fly off. It gave me the cold chills, mixed with relief; apparently, they did look after him, but I felt like I'd dodged a bullet.

I'd given Gwen my phone number in Minnesota, and she'd been calling me there, and before in Nebraska, quite a lot—

mostly to complain of the relatives, of the isolation, or the problems in simply dealing with the old man. He could be cantankerous when he wanted to. I recall one time at the new house
in Santee when an aid worker from one of the federal or tribal
agencies came out to give Elmer a quick checkup, he didn't want
to cooperate. I was standing by while Patti was arguing with him,
and I remember him saying, "I got nothing to do with them."

Patti had turned to me and said, "You see what I have to
put up with?"

"I'm not getting in the middle of this," I'd replied. There
was nothing I could do at that time, and I found it trying to hear
Gwen's litanies now, since I'd already been there, done that, and
had the T-shirt.

But before I completely leave the 2008 dance, there's one
more thing. I think monthly ceremony took place shortly after
the dance, or shortly before. I didn't go in, for I'd found myself,
once again on my own, stacking the grandfathers on their cradle
of logs after having asked Elmer how many to use. I piled up the
lengths of firewood as I'd done so many times in Santee into a
conical tower resembling a tipi, stuffing cottonwood bark and
cardboard underneath. The wind was quite high, and it was all
I could do to light one little scrap of tinder with my not-quite-
windproof lighter and set it in place. I was out of time; either
it got lit now or the rocks wouldn't be ready on time. But the
spirits must have been smiling on me for coming back as they'd
demanded. It only took that one try, and I watched as the tiny
flame ran its way up the paper, into the shredded back and onto
the pieces of cardboard, despite the prairie wind howling outside. I was fire keeper and doorman, which means I didn't sweat
that time. I could have gone in and steamed off, as they say, and
been OK for ceremony, but fire-keeping's hard work, and I didn't
want to have to stay up 'til 3:00 a.m. But the Hawk had gone in
and told me later it was probably a good thing I hadn't, because

Elmer said some things about me he probably wouldn't have had I been present; namely, he pointed to the huge pile of prayer ties I'd made in my seven years' absence and remarked, "There's people livin' on this reservation who ain't doin' that. He musta listened to me."

But to fill in the last blank, before winter set in, I was forced to change the plan, cancel the offer, and tell the Hawk via a phone message that he couldn't stay at my place any longer, to say nothing of all winter. The last straw was the afternoon he was all excited about his new girlfriend coming to pick him up. He'd been wearing me out with his small-minded worries, trying to guess her meaning from random statements, and started whining about my lack of sympathy (and interest). Then just ten minutes or so before she arrived, he cleared a space on the living room floor to do some push-ups. He did this by shoving a plugged-in radiant-style space heater up against a stack of vinyl records in their paper holders. The heater had a thermostat, and wasn't on at the time, but would be shortly. I just sat there and watched this. He did his push-ups, his girlfriend pulled up, and he was on with his shirt and out the door without even a glance at the fire hazard he'd just left behind.

I still said nothing, but that was it. I couldn't afford to have another house burn down. After the arson in northern Iowa, when I'd lost my cabin and trailer there, it was just too much of a risk. So after the message and a protesting response, I told him to come and pick up his things. There was a sizeable pile. Apart from the flute I'd bought him in Montana, the jacket he'd favored at the Salvation Army, and his clothes, there was the owl's feather from Rosebud. He came up driving her car late Monday morning, and that was the last of him I've seen. He did help me put up a fence but whined about having to work at assembling the gate hardware from boxes of parts. The farther we got from the Rainbow Gathering and sun dance, the less he wanted to work.

THOSE OF MY READERS WHO HAVE SUFFERED ALONG SO FAR MAY be grateful for an aside before I get to the spring of 2009. When I was in the little cabin in northeastern Iowa, after I'd begun drinking but before the spirits took my little shih tzu, I happened to be sitting up one night, doing some work with a sharp knife. Don't remember which knife or what the job was, but I slipped and drove the point an inch or so into the top of my right thigh. Try as I might, I could not get the bleeding to stop. It was a clean cut, and I hadn't hit any veins or arteries, but nothing would staunch it. I went through every bandage in my store-bought first-aid kit, and they stopped it for a bit, but as soon as I drove to a nearby campground for a shower, it started up again.

The second day, I was at my wits' end, when I recalled an episode from Santee. When I'd bought the little camper from Elmer and Patti and had remarked later that the stains on the ceiling looked like the roof leaked, Elmer had said, "Just take an' throw some tobacco up there, that'll stop any kinda leak." I also seemed to recall that the old-time Indians had used a mix of gunpowder and tobacco to clean out a wound so it wouldn't get infected. I had some iodine, so I ripped up one last bandage to go all the way around my leg, dismembered a whole American Spirit cigarette, slapped on the iodine, and applied the tobacco and tied it all up. It worked. It stung a bit, even through the iodine, but who cared? I'd had the leg of my jeans about soaked through to the knee by the time I got back from the shower. Grateful to Grandpa, once again.

CHAPTER 19

A Winter's Negligence

HOWEVER, BACK AT ELMER'S IN ROSEBUD, UNBEKNOWNST TO me, things had been going from bad to worse. Apparently, during November's monthly ceremony sweat, Elmer had told Dino to use only seven stones, and Dino took it upon himself to use the more usual twenty-one or twenty-two—anyway, many more than Grandpa had wanted. Gwen has since told me she feels that action led to the old man's second stroke. Also, Gilli and Webster and other relatives of Elmer's had come back and hung around all winter, using the ceremony house for a party house. They were drinking and taking apart some kind of capsules and snorting the contents. Gwen said that when she went in there to clean up, she found a lot of empty capsules. But the stroke was the worst. It left the old man paralyzed down his left side and unable to speak, at least for a while.

Meanwhile, I'd left Red Wing and was back in Nebraska for the winter. I'd left Gwen the Minnesota number and hadn't thought to get her an update. The relatives had threatened her in not-so-subtle ways—like Webster or another one of them honing a big knife while staring hard at her. She'd left and stayed at Nico's for a little bit, leaving the old man in Gilli's care, but then came back when that scene proved too chaotic. He'd been left lying in his own filth for a couple of days, unfed, and managed to say, when he could speak again, that Gilli had left the day before Gwen returned, and he'd said to another party who'd also decamped, "Just let him die in there."

Now that I recall, all this must have happened just before the holidays, since Gwen also told me that the old man had directed her to dress him in his best on Christmas. He was expecting some visitors, but no one came—none of his kids or even any of the local sun dancers came by or called.

Meanwhile, I was sending checks every month to Elmer, as I'd done in Santee years before I came to live there, through Nico. I had his address, and I thought I could trust him, as I didn't have Grandpa's. Only one of the checks got through. He never brought the rest over. Gwen later told me she'd seen one of them sitting on his kitchen table during the brief time she was there. At least he didn't try to cash them himself; he just spaced them off. Nico'd told me he'd be around, helping out, but I found out later that Grandpa had called him a bullshitter in ceremony, and that kind soured things between them. To make things even worse, Gilli had gotten drunk and wrecked the Dodge Ram pickup before the old man had even had it a year. Probably bullied the old man into giving him the keys, then went out and slammed it so hard into a pole, he bent the clutch housing.

So Gwen was there with Sage taking care of Grandpa pretty much by herself all winter, with no backup or relief. And he was paralyzed for the first month or so after the stroke. That is a damn hard road for anyone to have to walk, and a lot of people should have known better than to let it happen. I found out all of this in April of 2009 when I finally called from Nebraska.

During the call, I apologized for not giving her the Nebraska number; I also asked for a list of things they needed, which included some large flowerpots for her gardening and a new inset stove top for the trailer's kitchen. The old one had quit, and she'd been forced to prepare meals for three on a tiny hot plate for months. I had recently gotten a rather large tax refund, and with this I was able to buy a used 1995 Chevy pickup I'd seen at the dealership in Louisville. It's funny; I remember driving by the lot and seeing this green one out of all the others there. It turned out to be in good shape, very clean, and an automatic so I wouldn't be making the same mistake as with the Ram. I quickly managed to board all the animals, got the mail held, water off, and so on, and buy a tow bar and hitch from U-Haul.

This meant I had to make sure the Chev was towable with this particular unit and then drill four one-inch holes in the front bumper. I got a tight fit with the tow bar, but I was still pretty nervous about it, having never towed a vehicle for such a long distance. Four days before I set out, I put down my *pegi* pipe, so as to be clean when I picked up the real pipe, and prayed for a safe journey to help the *wicasa wakan* and that cook and her boy. Before making my prayers, however, there were a lot of errands to be run: going to Lincoln for the pots and soil, buying the titanium drill bit for the tow-bar holes, picking which instruments to bring (assuming I'd get any practice time), and laundry to wash, dry, and pack.

CHAPTER 20

Making Up for Lost Devotion

I REMEMBER GETTING OUT IN THE EARLY MORNING, SOON AFTER full light, and plugging my heavy power drill into an extension cord and feeling around on the inside of the curved face of the bumper to find the exact spots to drill. I had to mentally transpose the positions to the outside, then use a cold-steel chisel point to start the bit in so it wouldn't wander, and finish the drilling. The whole process of spacing, drilling, inserting the tow bolts, and tightening each one once the bar was set to the proper width took me a whole morning. But once it was in, I backed up the Chev, got out the box-cube van camper, lined 'em up, and the tow-bar hitch settled smoothly onto the ball mounted on the camper. Once the Chev was set in neutral, with the key in the on position to keep the power steering engaged, it towed easily.

It was a nerve-racking tow up to Rosebud, all the same. The weather was unseasonably hot for late May, more like the end of June. There was a hot wind blowing up out of the south with occasional gusts from the west. This made for a need to keep both hands on the wheel at all times and firm attention on the road. I had to take it slow as I left Wahoo and headed out into central Nebraska. To make things worse, a large road-construction project necessitated a long detour. I was forced to turn west after having detoured north, far to the south of where I usually would have. Suffice it to say bad roads and more detours along a strange route slowed me down considerably. Traveling as slowly as I was, I wouldn't have made the trip in one day anyhow, but this forced me to camp in a Super 8 for the night, after finally having gotten only as far north as O'Neill, Nebraska.

At my request, Gwen had hunted around the burned-out stove top and had gotten me the make and model. I'd made a few inquiries before I'd left, but no one had one in stock. Offers to order one in were no good, since my departure was by then imminent. But setting out along the long stretch of highway across northern Nebraska, I began to feel more optimistic. I happened to pass a large appliance store on the western edge of O'Neill, and although I'd just gotten under way in the cool morning, something told me to check it out. Luckily, their parking lot was big, encompassing two town lots or more, with an alley in back. It was easy to get in, turn around, and park without blocking anyone off, even with my long load. Gwen had told me she'd had to wait on Elmer hand and foot since his stroke, and for a moment, I considered purchasing a wheelchair and handicapped toilet accessories, but I held off. Lo and behold, they had a large selection of electric range tops, including the one I was after.

By nine thirty, I was off again and feeling great with the new stove stuck in the back of my camper. I also stopped at a Bomgaars for some chicken feed Gwen had requested. That went in underneath the stove. I might have put it all in the bed of the Chev, but I didn't want to increase the towed weight.

After a stop for lunch, I finally crossed into South Dakota. Another forty-five minutes of driving brought me up and over the long ridge—and with a stop to close the cattle gate behind me, I was back at Elmer's outfit.

I had called ahead on the morning I left Nebraska and again from the motel in O'Neill. Gwen had gotten Grandpa all dressed up in his best and out on the back porch in his wheelchair to greet me and to see the new truck. I pulled into the drive and circled around so the Chev was sitting right next to them.

I got out, came up and shook hands, responded to Elmer's *hau-hau-hau*, and greeted Gwen and Sage. Elmer's big, black three-legged shepherd mix, Lala, came up to say howdy too. I got out the keys and handed them to Elmer, saying, "I heard you didn't have a good truck, so I brought you this one." He took the keys from me gravely and shook my hand again. Then we all went inside.

Gwen had the coffee going, and as we sat around the kitchen table, she proceeded to fill me in on how things were going. Not all that well, which I'd already gathered. First off, I had to apologize for not thinking to give her the Nebraska phone number. Then she told me more about the relatives' misbehavior, her stay at Nico's, where she'd seen one of the checks I'd sent, and about the sweat where Dino had used too many rocks, and Grandpa's subsequent stroke. How hard it had been to be the solitary caregiver for a partially paralyzed and cantankerous elder—for months on end and without a relief. And then she broke down and started crying. I held her awkwardly for a bit, trying to soothe, but mostly just being there. And feeling mightily embarrassed and ashamed of myself for not calling sooner. I told her to take it easy, or something, I don't exactly remember, but that I would do anything I could to help.

Next, I went outside, got out my toolbox, and unbolted the tow hitch from the Chev's bumper. I borrowed the keys for a moment to make sure it would start and backed it next to the old man's bedroom window. Then I went off and parked my camper by the cookshack, unplugged my electrics from the on-board inverter, and plugged into the power pole. I hadn't had the foresight to leave my tools by the Chev, so after I toted the new stove over, still in its box, I had to walk back out for them. As I left, Gwen asked, "How long are you thinking of staying?"

"Until sun dance."

"You mean you're staying on?"

"Yeah."

The rest of the afternoon I busied myself with unloading the chicken feed and installing the new stove top. I recall dropping the tailgate of the Chev, once I'd got the tools over, and showing the new top to Gwen as I took it out of its box. The first step was to get it inside and get the power to the old one off. That done, I unscrewed the old top, disconnected it from the wiring harness, and took it out to the Dumpster. Had to do quite a cleanup job in the recess before I could even lift the new one over for a trial fit. Turns out it was somehow a little too big. Same model, same unit, but I had to get out my carpenter's rasp and Schrade folding knife and work the edges somewhat wider. Then I wired in the new one and powered it up for a test before screwing it in. Lo and behold, it worked, and Gwen was so happy to get rid of the miserable hot plate.

After that was done, I had time to say hello to Lala properly. As was the case the year before, there were a number of huge, blood-swollen deer ticks hanging off him. I vividly remember that big dog settling himself down in the drive, as I was on the front porch, and winking at me. I told him, "Lala, I know from last year you don't like to wear flea collars. What are we gonna do about all those ticks on you?"

Then I put away my tools and finished setting up the camper for an extended stay. I guess they were glad to have me; Gilli and others had been in the habit of showing up drunk and bullying money out of the old man and just generally carrying on as if it were their party house.

There was no such trouble the first few days I was there, but there were some amazing things. As I was walking out the front door the next morning, after coffee, to take stock of the toolshed, there was my forgotten rasp, right spang in the middle of the porch, as if someone had put it there. It really looked like a case of the spirits moving things. I told Gwen about the time I'd found the sage so long ago in Santee. And Lala showed up without a single tick on him. That dog was smart, smarter than some people I met out there.

The first few days out there were a little hard, though. Elmer was completely bedridden after his stroke. Even if Gwen had known to call Rick Two Dogs and ask for a long-distance doctoring, as Patti had done in 1999, it's doubtful that even the spirits could have done much for such an old man. It was painful to see him so reduced—but, for the most part, his mind was still clear. He still didn't seem to remember me from Santee, though, or the time in 2000–01.

His trailer was still where it had been the year before, and the ceremony house with the attached cookshack sat across the drive from it. About three hundred yards to the east were the four sweat lodges, with three benches and skulls and the eagle staff before the easternmost one. Just beyond them stood the sun-dance arbor. Going diagonally between the front door of the trailer and the arbor, the land fell off steeply into a deep gully. Just above the head of this, on the trailer side of the drive, there was first the little utility trailer that served as storage, and a little shade arbor next to this, with a metal-topped old desk for a workbench that had a vise bolted down on it. A few topless bureaus served for cubbies for the gas and oil, with a collection of threadbare tires along the fence to the south.

Just to the west of this, slightly closer to the cookshack than the trailer, was the chicken run and coop. The run was good sized, about twenty feet on a side, and Sage had charge of the chickens. He was very good at getting them fed and watered every morning, taking them their feed mixed with table scraps again in the evening and bringing in fresh eggs every day or so. There was a dozen or so hens, but no alarm clock (rooster).

Across the drive, in back of and slightly to the west of the big trailer, were a half dozen or so disabled vehicles, mostly pickups, including one Elmer had given to Gwen, which only needed a little work to get it going. A low fence line ran down from the main gate behind the trailer, and the trucks were parked along it. At the head of the row of trucks, but outside the parking area enclosed by the fence, was Elmer's school bus. On the other side of the fence, closer to the trailer, was Gwen's little camper-trailer. The Dumpster and main gate were about a hundred yards beyond the school bus, and from there, it was nearly a half mile to the crest of the ridge where the cattle gate was and the long, winding dirt road out to the highway.

The cattle gate was nothing more than two fence posts held together with strands of barbed wire, opened and closed with two loops of the same. It was opened and shut at the top and bottom of the near post by means of a long stick, which one used to lever the slack into the barbed wire and one had to slip off the top loop by hand. It scratched me good a few times before I took to carrying my elk-hide gloves everywhere I went.

All this was a tiny speck of habitation in the vastness of the South Dakota prairie. Off to the north and west were the main highway and the rez town of Parmelee, where we'd go to pick up the mail, do odds-and-ends shopping at the little trading post, and maybe buy some gas. But over it all were just hundreds and hundreds of miles of sky. That's how it looks once you get into the high plains. Don't know why—what interplay of land and atmosphere does it—but it's immense.

And there we all were. Word of my arrival spread pretty quickly, for the morning after my arrival, here comes Webster for a visit. Gwen later remarked he hadn't been up to see his dad for months. He approached me first, as I was finishing my morning coffee in my camper, with a request for some money to fix his cell phone. I refused, having been briefed by Gwen that he was following in Gilli's footsteps and had become a notorious drunk. He was back in about ten minutes, though—just came right up to the window where I had my little table and said, "My dad wants to see you." I reluctantly got out and went over to the trailer. It was a beautiful, bright spring morning, and the back door was open. Elmer was lying in his bed and told me to give Webster "some money so he could fix it, that phone." So I handed him a twenty. Web was so exuberant he thanked me, lifted up his dad's cap, and kissed him on the forehead. Then he was out the door and headed up the road to town, punching in a number, and talking on his phone as he went. I knew it was a low-down scam for drinking money from the first, but I still couldn't tell the old man no.

I had resolved, after talking to Gwen and hearing how badly his boys had been treating him, not to give any of them any-thing—and before the end of my first full day there, they'd already gotten around me.

There was a sweat coming up, and Jason (the camp crier from forever) was around, having either brought in or helped to bring in a load of firewood. I was surprised to see some of the old volcanic lava rocks from the year before were still being used. Most rocks, the ones that can be fired safely, can be used only once. They simply fracture under the stress of being cooled rap-idly, after being heated red-hot. But the lava rocks, I now recall, had been brought in 2001, and apparently some of them were still good. I'd been on a run into Mission (the largest town in Rosebud) a day or so after my arrival with Dino, and just as Gwen had detailed her problems with him to me, so he began catalogu-ing his with her.

I had gone with him, bringing a box of Elmer's socket wrenches to help him repair his vehicle, and we ended up stranded in Mission for most of the afternoon. On the way, he kind of surprised me by trying to build himself up in my eyes, saying he was "the eyes and ears" for Elmer. He shocked me by saying, "The spirits aren't done with that old man. He's gotta keep on doing ceremony for the people." This was impossible, of course, and hadn't been happening since Elmer's stroke and paralysis, which was at least partly due to Dino ignoring Grandpa's instructions for sweat. In hindsight, it's clear that Dino no longer felt himself as a follower of Elmer but as some kind of leader in his own right. He was maneuvering to get me into his flock.

Nonetheless, after the vehicle situation was resolved, I tried to make a truce. I told him that Gwen had told me how unhappy she'd been doing all the caretaking work on her own for so long, without a break, and mostly she wanted some positive recognition and support. "She wants you to at least come in and shake her hand," I said, "when you come by for a visit."

She'd told me in so many words she wanted that. And, upon our return, he did so. Gwen was a little taken aback. But this beginning was never built on any further—given his resentment of her "negativity," and her resentment of his neglect, and worse, there was no hope of a true reconciliation.

Once we'd gotten back, Dino immediately began loading up wood for the fire from the pile Jason had just finished stacking. We'd had a discussion, in which Jason informed me that Elmer had said that wood was to be used only for monthly ceremony sweat. Apparently, people were coming out to sweat at the new moon, even with no full ceremony afterward. I saw this and confronted Dino about it. He wouldn't listen, even when I told him Jason had relayed the word from Grandpa. He warned me off, saying Jason "was getting to think too much of himself," or words to that effect, and just kept loading up. I saw it was useless to insist and just went back to the trailer. That's kind of how things went that whole spring and summer. Dino was going to do things his way, regardless of what anyone, even Grandpa, had to say.

By the end of my second week in Rosebud, the weather began to change. Instead of dry, unseasonably warm temperatures, we began having a cool, rainy season. I was mostly helping Gwen with the shopping, minding Elmer when she took her infrequent trips to town, and helping get the trailer and its surrounds the way she wanted them. It became much cooler at night. I had to start using my electric and gas space heaters in the camper, and it rained almost every morning. I was also trying to get Elmer's collection of mowers, trimmers, and assorted gear working and in order.

Having arrived at the beginning of the last week in May, this cool and wet June weather was something of a surprise. However, before it set in, there seems to have been a somewhat longer period of warm and dry time than I've indicated. I was busy then, policing up the area around the sweat lodges, working on getting at least one of the Weedwackers working, and generally setting the place to rights. Gwen really wanted a garden, so I helped out with some fencing and gardening supplies, and together we worked on turning the bit of ground directly east of the trailer and in back, to the east of her camper, into tillable areas. It took something like two and a half weeks, but we got it done just before the end of planting time.

I had to drive a bunch of posts and stretch chain-link fence by hand, but she did all the gardening proper. I also made repeated trips to the local supply store / lumberyard in Mission and got her several hundred pounds of marble chips, so as to make a weedless space in front of her camper and a winding path through the garden in back. It was also then that I began stopping at a little hole-in-the-wall café there to pick up an order of chicken strips with fries for Grandpa's lunch. Gwen reported to me that once the fence was in and the garden planted, Elmer had remarked to her, "Looks like somebody's livin' here."

A while before the first garden was done, she started on the second plot, which was to be for more vegetables and corn. Over the hill to the east, about a mile off, was Irene Running and her outfit, still squatting in the old house where Elmer had raised his family before he moved to Santee—which was now providing a local haven for Gilli, Webster, and others. Two young men in their late teens began coming over, usually in the early afternoons, asking for work. I'd pay them so much per hour, and they'd dig and turn over the soil over until they got tired of it. Gwen used to talk to them, tell them they'd have to be strong and set an example as warriors for their people, but it turned out they were just doing it for drinking money. At least they got the second, larger plot finished and ready for planting. We really couldn't support them in this any longer, once she figured it out, but one day before the deal went down, they came over with guests of their own.

CHAPTER 21

Backdoor Man

ONE AFTERNOON, TWO ROLY-POLY PUPPIES ABOUT TEN OR twelve weeks old followed them over. One was black, and one looked like the shepherd mix, Hampa, Sage had had the year before. Hampa wasn't around now. Late in the winter, the last of the relatives finally left. These were Anthony Running, who was called Iktomi, and his woman. They had been very abusive, even threatening toward Gwen, but when it came time to leave, they begged her for gas money. Gwen didn't have much to give; Grandpa was so afraid of being robbed he was keeping a really tight hold on the purse strings. But she gave them a single dollar. That night was the last time anyone saw Hampa. Gwen told me they'd figured that the departing couple had called him into their vehicle and dumped him somewhere. Up to that point, that was the worst thing I'd ever heard.

Sage was inconsolable. She told me he was crying, going on about losing his only friend, and imagining the dog's distress: "We gotta pray for her, Mom!"

"It was pitiful," Gwen said with a sigh, shaking her head.

Turns out the main reason Anthony stayed on for so long was that there was a felony warrant out for his arrest in Minnesota. Not long afterward, we heard that he'd been picked up and was spending the foreseeable in the correctional facility in Stillwater, Minnesota. Couldn't have happened to anyone more deserving. Ordinarily, I hate the thought of any Indian rotting in a white man's prison; the only thing the first Indian prisoners were guilty of was fighting for their homeland and their people's freedom against inexorable tyranny. A lot of them were lied to—probably all, really—assured they'd be removed to a new reservation, and then those deemed hostile were imprisoned.

But these two puppies seemed like they belonged with us, so I asked one of the guys if they'd sell them. The answer was yes, and when I handed over a ten, thinking it was for one of them, he waved away my offer of another ten, saying it was enough for both. So Sage got the one that resembled Hampa, and I got the other. The little black one I named Mahto, which is "bear" in Lakota. I had to go to town and buy some puppy chow, in addition to the dog chow I was already getting for Lala and the yellow one who came around sometimes. I also had to keep watch over the morning feedings, since Hokshila was a very aggressive eater. I had to space the bowls and hubcaps far apart until the pups learned that their food was for them and Lala's was for him. In a week or so, Sage and I made a run down to the vet's in Valentine and got them their checkups and shots. I remember Sage and I had lunch at Subway and generally had a good time.

Back at the ranch, Gwen and I visited some more. She told me how little she'd been seeing of anyone, except for Lorna and Gorgie, the senior lady sun dancers. She said she'd been promised a raise in the little she was getting since Elmer's stroke. She'd been chief cook and bottle washer from before then, despite all the grief from the relatives, but after the stroke and her return, it had been round-the-clock invalid care. The promised raise had never materialized, and she was barely getting enough to make ends meet, even with what Elmer gave her from his own personal funds for shopping. I'd started making some grocery runs, which

began turning into a regular weekly thing, including the basket
of chicken strips for his lunch. Her macaroni hot dish with cheese
and green enchilada sauce was a treat on cool, wet evenings.

One day, she suggested I take Elmer out for drive in the new
pickup. The next morning, after I breakfasted in my camper and
fed the dogs, she got Grandpa dressed in his black jeans, shirt,
cowboy boots, and black leather vest. It was something of a late
start to the day; we didn't get away until after lunch. Our goal
was twofold: to get the pickup registered in Elmer's name while
getting him out of his room for a while so Gwen would have a
chance to clean up and deodorize in there. After a few unfortunate spills, the carpet was beginning to smell. The weather was
clear and warm for a change, and we had little or no trouble at
the courthouse in Winner, although there was a question as to the
validity of the signature; his son Norman's name had come up in
connection with some dubious registrations. I say *we*, although of
course it was I who went inside and up the two flights of stairs to
the Taxes and Vehicles desk.

I remember telling the lady, "This vehicle's a gift from me
to Elmer; if you need him, he's outside sitting in it right now."
But they knew who Elmer was, and all I had to do was run the
form back out to him, have him sign it, and then pick up the
new South Dakota license plates. I'd taken off the bumper-hitch
plates, so the front plate-holder was unobstructed, but I had to
borrow a screwdriver from a merchant on the town square. Being
a tribal vehicle now, no proof of insurance was required, as the
tribal nations are not subject to every state law.

Then we set out south through town, and this is where our
trouble began. I had a new road atlas, but I'd never taken this
route to Valentine before and was unsure of the way. We stopped
at the first little town, at a three-way intersection, to ask directions, went down the wrong leg of road, had to go back and ask
again. Elmer started to lose patience with me, or perhaps it was

the effort of sitting upright for so long. "You a bullshitter!" he exclaimed.

"No, I'm not, Elmer. I told you I never went this way before! I didn't say I knew it!"

We finally got on the right road, but it was a long drive. Too long for the old man. I remember I was getting uptight already with not knowing the way, when he said he couldn't sit upright anymore; he had to lie down in the backseat. I got him stretched out back there, but it wasn't easy. He seemed to weigh so much more that he appeared to. A gravel road cut across our highway just there, and as I was trying to wrestle the old man into a comfortable position, a UPS truck pulled up at the farmhouse across the way. I briefly considered asking the driver for help, but he was out and away too fast. I must have tugged too hard at some point, 'cause Grandpa yelled, "Easy, goddamn it! I'll bust them glasses for you!" Referring to my shades.

"I'm sorry! I was tryin' to do it easy!"

A few miles down the road, still well shy of Valentine, I could tell Grandpa was starting to have a hard time; I could hear him groan as he tried to shift himself into a more comfortable position. I began driving as fast as I dared, a little more over the limit than usual. I finally recognized the main drag and grocery store of a little town I'd been through before and knew we weren't too far from Valentine. Before we got there, though, we had to cross a little stretch of upland, as the land was rising to the long Pine Ridge. Just as afternoon was becoming evening, Elmer let out a particularly loud gasp. Sounded like he was in some pain, but I didn't know what I could do to help. In the next moment, seeming to have come from nowhere, there was a little black-tailed deer standing by the side of the road. It was a buck; I remember seeing its odd-looking rack. It was as if Elmer's distress had summoned one of his helping spirits, as the black-tailed deer is listed as such, with its appropriate ties, on the sheet of instructions for monthly ceremony and sun dance. It seemed to be waiting for us. Standing stock-still until we'd passed, I saw in the rearview it had bounded across the road directly behind us and was quickly lost to view.

Grandpa seemed to get more comfortable after that. At least he was quieter. I don't think we talked at all the rest of the trip, but after what seemed to me like forever, we were through Valentine, back in Rosebud, and finally got back to Mission, where at his request I stopped for a basket of chicken strips, and we were soon home.

"Did you boys have a good ride?" inquired Gwen as we helped Elmer out of the pickup and into his wheelchair. Elmer just grunted, and I said, "Not exactly," and proceeded to give her an account of the journey, including my fear that he was gonna die on me and I'd be held responsible for it. That'd been on my mind at one point, just before the deer showed up, when I realized we were off in the middle of nowhere and far from any help, at the least the conventional kind.

After that, I confess I was a little shy of hanging out with the old man, at least for any length of time. A routine request for the keys to the pickup was invariably met with the peevish injunction to: "Come right back! Goddamn it! Don't you go off nowheres!"

I began to realize, and Gwen confirmed, that the stroke had altered his personality. Once before our road trip, Gwen had encouraged me to go back and just to sit with the old man. I did this, lit us up a pair of cigarettes, didn't say too much, and just sat looking out the window. But I could tell by his increasingly agitated body language that he couldn't remember me and was unsure about this great big *wasicu* hanging in his bedroom.

June continued cool and wet. During a solo trip into Valentine, I remember seeing one of the local ranchers in his high boots and jean jacket walking along on the other side of Main

Street with a big smile on his face. The weather certainly boded
well for good crops and low feed prices. I was in town to pick up
some things that couldn't be found in Mission, fill up the mowers' gas cans, and do some pokin' around on my own. The chairs
around the kitchen table were all mismatched and uncomfortable,
so after checking off the items on Gwen's list, I wandered over
to the antique and thrift shop. I found a nice set of six kitchen
chairs, and after calling the seller, I managed to negotiate a decent
price for them. After filling up, I once again stopped in Mission
for a chicken-strip basket and got back around lunchtime. After
returning the keys to Elmer and waiting until someone was with
him as he ate, I took the old chairs out to the ceremony house.
The new ones looked good, and it was also about this time I
managed to fix the leaky hot-water line in to the washer in the
hallway. The leak was rotting out the floorboards beneath and
into the hall.

This may seem to be getting awful close to tooting my own
horn, but all I'm really trying to do is tell what happened.

On my next trip into Mission, I got a new dryer; the old one
had a set of bearings that were shot, and every time we used it,
it set up the most ungodly howling screech. It made me want to
shoot it. I asked Gwen how long it had been doing that, and she
replied, "All winter!" Taking everything together, she and Sage
had been having a pretty bad time of it. A lot of the sun dancers dropped off gifts for Sage the previous summer, and they
deserve credit for that. Gwen also informed me that the relatives
had rarely cleaned up after Elmer, or indeed at all, in the house.
The place was a pit by the time she'd returned from Nico's. Also,
Elmer's room stank of urine—the carpets and the blankets and
particular, and the rainy weather was bringing it to the fore.
One of the things I'd been sent for was a carton of Febreze anti-
stank juice.

In addition to everything else, the old man would be awake
at all hours, and Gwen was rarely getting a good night's sleep.
One story I heard several times was when Grandpa awakened her
at 1:00 a.m., needing someone to light his cigarette. She'd gotten
up off the couch, gone back and lit it for him, and he'd taken one
drag and stubbed it out. He'd been pretty peremptory up until
that point, even yelling at Sage once and calling him a "little
monkey," but at that crack, and at the cigarette incident, Gwen
had yelled right back, demanding that he be respectful to her son
and that he treat her with some respect too, or she was leaving.
That brought him around. He was nicer after that, but I had to
stand my own ground with him once also. He began speaking
abusively to me, kinda snarling when I asked him for the keys
to the Chev one morning, and I got tired of it. "Look, Elmer!"
I exclaimed. "I brought that pickup for you, you got that title,
and all I'm tryin' to do is help out with it! I don't ever go runnin'
around in it, and I always bring it right back and park it right
there where you can see it. You don't need to yell at me and call
me a bullshitter when I'm doing everything I can around here!"

That made him get quiet. Gwen and I talked it over later on.
That's when I heard what came after the cigarette incident. "He
never would apologize," she said. "But the next day, he called me
back there and gave me a pack of his cigarettes. And he told Sage
that after he was gone, he'd always be around as Sage was growing up, looking out for him."

I've neglected to mention that at the previous year's sun
dance, the spirits had given Sage his Indian name, Wanbli
Hokshila Ishnala Mani, or Little Eagle Boy That Walks Alone.

As for Dino, he wasn't around much, but I'd mentioned to
him during our afternoon in Mission that I'd like to get up on the
hill that year, and he hadn't forgotten. I never did get up there;
between the relatives' craziness, Elmer's illness, and all the work
that had to be done for sun dance, which all fell to me at first, I

never got the time. Sure wish I had. Dino also told me that Elmer had said to him, "Get the campin' area good, and look after them outhouses; there's gonna be a lotta people here for my funeral."

After the puppies had been around for a few weeks, there was a combination sun-dance meeting and wood-cutting party. The puppies and Lala had seemingly worked out a treaty of nonaggression, and as soon as I'd gotten my camper set up, Lala took up station underneath. He'd dug himself a little hollow right under the rear of my van and stayed there every night. The puppies would come and snuggle up next to him, and it was a sight to see them all get up in the morning. For some dog reason, when Lala was yawning, the little ones would come up and stick their heads into his open mouth. They'd do it other times too, and Gwen and I mentioned how weird it looked.

In late June, a party of sun dancers came in from points out of state, and we went out with about a dozen guys and a couple of chainsaws in the chill mist that was coming down. I had mentioned to Dino about wanting to go up on the hill, and now I repeated the same intention to a nice guy I'd seen many times before at sun dance, Steve from Indiana. I was riding in his Suburban with a couple of other guys and a little girl who was one of the kids Dino had adopted.

Another of Gwen's grievances against Dino was that he'd had a good job with the tribe but quit it several months earlier, saying that he was done cooking and was going to come out and help Elmer more or less full-time. Well, he'd rarely come by at all, but the one time he came with all his kids for a visit, they'd left the place trashed, food wrappers and drinks all over the place. They didn't throw a single thing in the trash. I didn't see that, so I can't say, but on our return trip with a load of wood in the back, the little *wincincala* got out in a hurry and ran for the trailer. Steve immediately saw that she'd spilled her Coke all over the seat and the inside of the door. "Little bailout!" he exclaimed.

Nonetheless, we had a good sweat that day and a satisfactory sun-dance meeting afterward. Later on, Jason and I were working on one of Grandpa's pickups that still sorta ran, changing a tire. We'd had to use a precarious arrangement of cinder blocks and logs to get the vehicle high enough to change the tire, and Steve happened to be standing by. We got the old tire off, and he suddenly warned us against getting our hands too far underneath. Jason was muttering something about this not being the first tire he'd changed when the supports gave way, and the truck came down in a hurry. Steve was exercised about it, saying, "You can't tell me there's no such things as spirits!" He was referring to the lucky timing, since we'd kept our hands on the job after he'd spoken but got them out just before the collapse.

By the next day, it was just the four of us again. I spent the first part of the morning on that most unglamorous of the old Indian ways, cleaning out the sweat lodges. Dumping the grandfather rocks with respect in the large half-moon shape off to the west of the woodpile, sweeping out the lodges afterward, and policing up the fire-pit area. Back in Santee, Elmer had always kept the area around the lodges really neat. There were benches for the participants, made of two-by-tens nailed onto lengths of cottonwood trunks, empty coffee cans for cigarette butts, and the pairs of deer antlers, used by the person sitting directly to the left as one entered, nearest the door, to lift the red-hot stones. These were tied together with leather string and hung up on a nearby pole. They had to be; otherwise, the mice would eat them, or some hungry *sunka* (dog) would carry them off. Nothing special happened this time, though; no bundle of sage appearing mysteriously, but I was on the lookout for something, whatever it might be. In his famous novel *Little Big Man*, Thomas Berger kinda hits the nail on the head at least once when he sums up the difference between the white and red worlds: As to the Indians, he wrote,

"They wasn't walking around expecting to be swindled; on the other hand, they was always ready for a miracle."

It's sad how Christianity and most of the other monotheistic religions have robbed man and nature of their miraculousness and placed it out of reach in something theologians are pleased to call "the Godhead." Ever since man was placed at the center of creation, thereby thinking the earth was his to do with as he pleased, we've had inquisitions, holy wars, jihad, genocide, and the ruination of the planet. Indians had plenty of wars, but not with body counts in the thousands and hundreds of thousands, and not because of religious differences. I've heard a recording of one Native man saying that before Columbus got here, from the Arctic to Amazonia, it was all one religion, just with regional variations, which apparently troubled no one.

I recall now that there was another presence at Elmer's trailer whom I've neglected to introduce: a little gray-and-white, half-grown, half-starved, half-wild kitten that spent most of its time hiding under the porch, but would come out up on the carpeted ramp for a lie-down in the afternoon sun. We used to feed it by setting a bowl of cat food on the handrail, about two-thirds of the way up, just outside the living room window. It was very shy, but once it got used to them, it would come out and play with Mahto and the other puppy, whom Sage had named Dakota. They sure had some good tussles!

Lala got around amazingly well for a three-legged dog. I tried to keep him from jumping the fence and running the neighbor's cattle, but the herding instinct was too strong, and Grandpa didn't believe in tying up dogs. I had a lot of respect for that dog after the tick-disappearing incident, but I was afraid he was starting to teach the pups to run the livestock. I didn't want the drunken rancher shooting at them too. This was the same guy who'd come roaring into sun-dance camp on his little four-wheeler, charged into the trailer, and done some yelling at

Grandpa because someone had left the gate open. Fortunately, he wasn't around much.

One who did put in an appearance soon after the wood-cutting party was Gilli. He had a bad habit of back-dooring his way in, avoiding Gwen and myself, and badgering the old man about this and that in Lakota. He was usually after money. This time, he showed up with his blonde *wasicu win* and three or four white guys he'd convinced he was a *wicasa wakan*. He was putting one or more of them up on the hill, just went over to the sweat lodges without stopping in, and started up a fire. We heard later on that he wouldn't bring in his own *canunpa*, probably because of the blood he'd spilled and the life he'd taken. We had to watch him, because things would go missing after he'd leave. It had come up at the sun-dance meeting that we'd have to ask all the sun dancers who attended to do a phone tree to all the rest, to let them know the date for purification.

This was necessary because Gilli had stolen Grandpa's notebook from the previous year with all the names, addresses, and phone numbers in it. We began hearing from people who said Gilli had called and told them the date was some nine days or so after the date Elmer had already set. He did this, obviously, to lure people away from Elmer's bona fide sun dance and get them to come to his sham one. He'd already had one in the Black Hills shut down, but I guess that wasn't enough. We couldn't call people and correct his misinformation, since we didn't have the book.

Gwen had also accused him of deliberately putting bedbugs in the living-room sofa. She described how at one time she'd been lured away from the trailer to the ceremony house by Gilli's woman, leaving him alone with Elmer. She got suspicious, raced back over, and surprised Gilli in the act of doing something strange. She said he'd looked startled by her reappearance and had some kind of trash like cotton ticking in his hand, which he'd promptly shoved out of sight. The fact remains that there were no bedbugs in the place before this incident, but there were plenty after. Elmer was getting bit, Gwen was, and every time I lay down or sat there for any length of time, I was. It's like some-one poking you with a hot needle.

But I must retrace my narrative a few weeks and go back to the third week I was there; Elmer's birthday was coming up, and Gwen reminded me that he was feeling pretty depressed about that time. He kept saying he was gonna kick the bucket and telling her she'd have to put on a dress and sit in the ceremony house, 'cause that's where his funeral was going to be. And he was talking about a spot way out past the edge of the camp-ground for a burial. Gwen was still doing most of the caretaking, while I fetched in groceries and supplies and tended to mower maintenance out in the toolshed. But one morning, she said he'd been talking that way, and "I had to use my best scolding voice and tell him, 'Grandpa, I'm planning your birthday party right now, and I don't have time for a kick-the-bucket party.' And he got this funny look on his face, and said 'OK, then!'"

We got word that one of his grandsons had just graduated on the high school honor roll, so I went to the trading post just south of Mission and got a ribbon shirt for honoring and a nice card to send to the young man, to be signed by Grandpa. Gwen and Gorgie were doing the heavy party planning, but as usual, it was Gwen who gave me my marching orders to go to Buche Foods, the big grocery store in Mission, and pick up the birthday cake, with a nice photo of him done in frosting. Plus lots of pop, chips, can-dles (but not the full eighty-eight), and cards for us to give him.

When the day came, lots of people came, a couple of his boys, and a drum group. I wish I could tell more about the details of the event, but when you're involved in the legwork, the details sometimes drown out the memories of the big picture. I recall a bunch of us singing "Happy Birthday" and that the weather was still cool and wet, which meant there wasn't much of an opportunity for folks to sit outside at the picnic tables and socialize. So it didn't go on for as long as it might have.

Anyhow, a day or so later, here comes Gilli with his gaggle of dupes again, helping themselves to the wood we'd cut, not asking for permission, not even a greeting. We judged it best just to let it be, since he wasn't coming up to the trailer and hassling the old man. No, now I recall he did come in, ignoring Gwen and myself, and went back to see his dad. They conversed in Lakota for a while. He must have fed Elmer some falsehood, for I can't believe Elmer would have agreed to what went on. Anyway, Gilli came back out front and tried his best to be civil. Knowing him as we did, we knew it was just pretense, and Gwen ducked out so she wouldn't have to shake hands with him. I was nearer to the door and couldn't escape. That day, I got a little understanding of how some medicine men can tell the state of a person through the handshake. I felt as if my hand had just gotten something nasty on it. I couldn't help it; once he'd turned away, I reenacted the scene from *Thunderheart* and rubbed my hand against my jeans, trying to get it off. So, off he goes, gets these guys off the hill, through sweat, and they take off. We found out later he'd used some *hanblechiya* sites over on Irene's land. When she found out about it, she was mad as a wet hen. "I don't want no *wasicu* goin' up on the hill on my land!" For once, I agreed with her.

I remember being in the little backyard, between the rows of vehicles and Gwen's trailer, when these guys came up with Gilli to head out. I just watched as one of them waved to me. I wanted so badly to warn them. They seemed sincere, but something held me back. Perhaps a smidge of the wisdom of the old ways: Let each one find his or her own path. Besides, anything I'd say would only be more talk. No reason they should listen to me. I could only offer up a quick prayer that they'd come to a good understanding soon about whom they were really dealing with.

After my own first impressions of Gilli in Santee, plus what Gwen told me Elmer had said about him, I found him the kind of guy I wouldn't want to have my back to. Apparently, there'd been a knife fight the previous autumn—alcohol was involved—and he'd stabbed Norman and Webster. Iktomi, too, had shed the blood of a relative, or so I'd heard, and Elmer had forbidden the two of them to ever sun dance again.

This was hard to reconcile with what Elmer had said to me back in the spring of 2001: "Gilli's gon' be a medicine man," he'd remarked to me out of nowhere, as if he was mystified by it. Of course, the spirits had told him that. He couldn't understand it at the time, I guess, but now it was coming true, but not in a good way.

It had been some weeks now, since the two young men had stopped coming over from Irene's to help work on the second garden. I was still busy every day, when I wasn't on a run into Mission or Valentine. After having changed the mowers' oil and plugs and gotten them running, it was still too wet most days to do much mowing. So I built a frame out of two-by-fours, scooped out a depression in front of her little camper, laid down a sheet of plastic first, and filled the space with the white marble chips. That's how Gwen wanted it. I also built a similar frame for the front of the big trailer, where she planted flowers.

One sunny day, Gorgie had come by to spend the day with Elmer, and Gwen and I made a run down to the greenhouse in Valentine. In addition to the plants she bought, I got some green iron fence posts and wire fencing to stretch by hand around her main garden in back. She went to town on it in more ways than one too, and with all the rain, it wasn't long before she had a garden full of growing veggies, with corn coming up in the other plot.

As to the critters, we needn't have worried about Lala. He took the pups' frolicsomeness in stride, even when they joined him under my camper every night. I had to get back in the habit of carrying a little plastic bag for cleanup around in my back pocket and tried to get Sage to do the same, since one of the dogs was his. He seemed to regard them both as his, as I found out a little later on, but I was planning to take black Mahto back home with me and hope he'd fit in with my colony of shih tzus.

The weather was beginning to warm and dry up, and I was finally able to mow around the mobile home and out in the north parking area, past Gwen's camper, but I was saving the huge camping and parking area west of the arbor for a little later. Elmer had one riding mower, but it needed a lot of work. Once I'd drained out the old oil, I sharpened the blades, changed the plug, and got new oil in. It seemed to go all right for a while. But we were going to need more for the ten-plus acres that needed to be done.

So one sunny morning, Elmer and I made a run into Valentine. I have to admit I was starting to get a little spooked hanging out with the old man. Ever since the stroke, there was no telling what might set him off into a fit of temper. It made me wish I'd spent my time, the year before, in Rosebud instead of playing around in Wyoming at the Rainbow Gathering. But if I hadn't headed out across the divide, I'd never have found that buzzard's wing (which made a dandy sun-dance fan) or encountered Morningstar. As for her, I'd tried to keep in touch by phone and had gotten through once, but then the number I had for her began ringing at some other people's place, and directory assistance was no help in locating her. I'd prayed for her good health and help, since she'd asked me to, but getting in touch was a no-go.

Anyway, our trip to Valentine was unmarred by any outbursts. The weather had resumed cool and wet, I got the groceries Gwen had asked for and picked up some smokes for us all. Then Elmer and I stopped at a large farm-supply store. There was a large scoop shovel hanging on a rack outside, and he said I should get it, since we had nothing but a small, flat-bladed spade for cleaning out the lodges and the fire pit. I got it and came back out, and he gave me the thumbs-up. Then he told me to drive over to another such place, the Bomgaars on the edge of town. At first I'd misinterpreted his directions and parked at a feed store, but he told me to park across the street. There were a number of new riding mowers there, and I asked him what he wanted, but he clammed up on me. It was getting kind of frustrating dealing with him for another reason; when he tired of a subject, or forgot about it, or thought I should know the answer already, there was no getting another word out of him.

So I checked out the lineup of mowers without really being sure what I was doing there. I figured this must be it, just as a salesman came out, and we began the dickering on the smallest of them. It was the only one that would fit in the back of the Chev. I ended up getting it, and this seemed to satisfy the old man. There was no question it was needed, and I was happy I'd solved the small puzzle he'd posed.

Well, we got back after the stop in Mission for the inevitable chicken-strip basket, and Gwen and I loaded him into his wheelchair and got his boots off and his moccasins on and back into bed. Gwen helped him eat while I unloaded the mower by driving a little ways into the steep-sided gully, dropping the tailgate onto the slope, and driving the mower off. Again, I was thinking, for such a slight man, Elmer was heavy! It was all I could do on subsequent trips to get him from his chair into the pickup seat without dropping him. I couldn't help giggling a bit as Dave Ross's words came back to me: "He broke our medicine man!" But if Gwen had been having to lift him for cleaning, bathing, and dressing all winter, it was no wonder she was in shape.

It was about this time, near the end of spring, that a fellow named Vern Yellowhawk showed up. He was a tall Indian guy, obviously, from Oak Creek, another little rez town. He was fluent in Lakota and said he wanted to help out. By now, the drier, warmer weather was getting more usual, so with the new mower, I was starting on the large camping and parking areas. Vern seemed pretty willing at first, seemed like a nice guy at first. He'd spend hours mowing; as long as he got to ride the new one. I noticed right away that he was agreeable enough for the less taxing chores but more unwilling to set his hand to anything too much like drudgery. Turns out, Dino had recruited him to come help out, and this was one more bad move by Dino. Initially, it was hard for me to accept Gwen's overwhelmingly negative opinion of Dino, but his backing of Yellowhawk started the tide turning. Grandpa didn't want him around, had even whacked Vern with his cane one morning when he was out in his wheelchair.

After he'd been around a couple of weeks, I wanted to go to an art show and sale at Sinte Gleska University one evening in Mission. Vern wanted to go too, and I noticed as we left that he was holding a little parcel in a tightly folded paper bag. After we got away from the place, out on the highway, he began begging me to allow him to drive, saying, "I haven't got to drive anywhere in a long time!" I was very unwilling to let anyone else drive the Chev, since I'd had a particularly hard time getting the keys from Elmer that evening. I'd had to explain that all I wanted to do was to go to the art show, and he'd finally agreed.

Vern kept up his whining, however, and I finally, reluctantly, agreed. Immediately, he began driving away from Mission, saying he just wanted to visit some friends over by Saint Francis, and it would be only a minute. We finally got to where he was going, and he disappeared into a little BIA/HUD prefab with an overgrown yard and driveway. He came back out a few minutes later, minus his little parcel, and so did a young NDN man, dressed gangsta-style—big wide shorts, tank top, and sneaks. This one gave me a thumbs-up and a big smile. I waved back, not liking the feel of the situation at all.

I demanded the keys back from Vern as soon as he got back to the Chev, and I drove us to the show. But en route, he complained loudly to me about horses running loose on the road, saying they killed drivers, to distract me from what he was doing. On the way to the show, I gave him some grief about having a destination but not telling me about it and saying he only wanted to drive. That evening was the last time we saw some of the DVD movies, mostly Westerns, that I'd brought for Grandpa to watch. It was obviously (in hindsight) a barter for drugs or *pegi*, but we didn't figure this out 'til later.

At the art show, I bought some hair-pipe beads, some sinew, and a wonderful ceramic miniature of a bear's head from one of the artists. Then we went back before full dark, and I gave the keys back to Elmer. After I'd told Gwen about Vern's mysterious behavior, she started calling around and finally found a woman over in Oak Creek who knew him. "Don't let him in," the woman said. "He's a liar and a thief!"

Before we detected the theft, however, and Gwen made the call, there was pressure from Dino to keep Vern around. After we gave him the boot, Dino told me to my face that he was going to be back around. Dino was getting more and more into building a base of followers and doing things his own way to set himself up as a sun-dance leader. Jason had told me, earlier, "Dino puts himself above the pipe."

Notwithstanding this, I have to give him credit for a couple of things. He reminded us of something Grandpa had said—since monthly ceremony was no longer being held, we should all pick up our *canunpas* at the time of the new moon and pray then. "That's as close as we can come to ceremony."

I'd also informed him of my intention to go up on the hill, and he said he'd put me up there sometime that spring. But it never seemed like the opportunity arose. I'd gotten a big blanket, a new knife, bucket, and ladle, and had even gotten all the ties and flags made, but one thing and another kept me hopping all the time. First, the wet weather prevented any such plans, then mowing and the monkey business with Vern, since I was unwilling to leave Gwen and Grandpa alone with him. And the basic, routine grocery shopping and giving Gwen a break from tending to the old man when she wanted to be the one to go to town.

However, a little over a month into my stay, Dino did present me with a beautiful gift. He asked me if I had an eagle feather, since you needed one to go up on the hill. I told him no, I didn't have one. He'd said, later on, he had a feather ready to go for me, but that was it. We didn't see him for a good while after that, and turns out he was waiting for me to give him the word, whilst I was waiting for him to bring the feather. One day he came over with it and presented it to me: "In honor of all the work you're doing here." Wow. Gwen had encouraged me to just load up my pipe and *opagi* Elmer, but it never felt right to me. Perhaps I missed a great opportunity, but on the other hand, I didn't miss the feather. I had to accept it on that basis; it's one thing I still have to respect him for.

CHAPTER 22

Sylvan

IT WAS, HOWEVER, A SHORT TIME BEFORE THIS, THE WEEK after we'd given Yellowhawk the old heave-ho, that a refugee from Irene's showed up at our door. His name was Sylvan, and he was originally a native of Rosebud who'd been living in Gordon, Nebraska. He'd had a job over in eastern Iowa at one of the kosher meat-packing plants that had been closed down by the feds after they'd hired an abundance of undocumented aliens. He'd been living over at Irene's, where he told us he'd been offered a place to stay, but his stuff would turn up missing if he went anywhere. There were meals available, in theory, but the immediate family ate first, and sometimes there was nothing for anyone else. Gwen seemed to think he was OK and helped kit him out with deodorant, soap, razor, and such. I also did what I could to help him. Sylvan would come over, usually in the evenings, sit and talk, and do some artwork. I began asking him to do a series of drawings, on a one-at-a-time sort of basis. I'd pay him twenty dollars for a single full-page drawing, in colored pencil.

Gwen would invite him to supper, and we'd sit and talk a bit over coffee. His vehicle was broken down, and he was worried about his family back in Gordon. He had an unemployment check coming every week, but it was sometimes delayed.

One afternoon, when I'd done all the mowing I could, I was sitting in the mobile home. Gwen was at her computer at the kitchen table, and Sage was off outside somewhere. It was the middle of June, and I got up to take a peek outside. That was the thing about living way out on the rez—with the kind of relatives we had to deal with, you could never feel completely safe. There was always the possibility that someone or other would show up drunk, or that Gilli would come in on the QT, park out of sight, and be in the back door badgering the old man for money. Gwen had remarked that she'd found several hundred dollars hidden in Grandpa's hung-up clothing one time when she'd gone to do his laundry. Sylvan had told us that Gilli and Irene were doing their version of monthly ceremony and that he "didn't think it was right for someone to be praying with the pipe one day and be out in the backyard with a beer in his hand the next." So, looking out the window to be keeping an eye on things, I saw a sight that made me whisper hurriedly to her, "Gwen! You gotta come over here and see this!" She came and started laughing. The little cat and one of the pups'd begun playing with a length of loose carpet that the dogs had been using for a chew toy. It was just nailed onto the front porch, but they'd pulled three or four feet of it loose, in a long string, and were lying there together, all tangled up in an unimaginable mare's nest, looking as happy as clams. I wish I'd had a camera, but there wasn't one in the house.

By now, it was getting to be too hot to work all through the day. I'd get up early, a little before dawn, go down to the trailer, dislodge Lala from the front porch, where he'd ensconce himself before I got there, and, usually, have to knock and rouse Gwen from the couch. Then I'd start the coffeemaker, get some food, and start on whatever work was on hand for the day. By this time, I'd begun the long process of repairing the stringers and crutches comprising the arbor. Unlike the one in Santee, the uprights were to be painted all white, so I'd gotten a couple of gallons of latex outdoor paint while on a run to Mission. Before the painting could start, though, there were several uprights to replace, some still needed the bark stripped off, and the stringers had to be replaced once the crutches were finished. By *replaced*, I mean that they were next to their appropriate crutches and needed to be put back in place. This was lucky, as there was no nearby stand of ash trees out on the open prairie. Santee had been all wooded lowlands.

I'd finished the mowing since Vern left, and when I'd asked Elmer how he'd wanted the arbor painted, he'd said, "Just white." He'd always been spare with his words, but now he was positively taciturn. If no one was in back with him and he needed or wanted something, he could still set up a yell, as Gwen knew all too well, and he never failed to growl at me when I asked him for the pickup keys: "And don't you go runnin' round with it! You come right back, goddamn it!" But his instructions were few, and Gwen told me he was slipping off into some space where he didn't distinguish between then and now or here and elsewhere. More than once, Gwen had mentioned how he'd called her into the bedroom and asked her where the trees were; there were trees to the east, to the west of his old place, where Irene and them were now, but not here.

"It's like he's slipping into another world, kind of," she said. "When he does that, I can't get him to talk to me about what's really going on. There was one time when he wanted to move the whole trailer back there. I said, 'Grandpa, I don't think your old trailer is gonna take another move.'" She said these lapses had started after his stroke and had begun to increase in frequency.

Then there was the time Elmer told me he had a whole other outfit, just up the road. He told me he had another house, with another closet hung with his clothes, boots, and tools. I was back in the bedroom when he said this, standing in for Gwen, and he seemed angry when I appeared bewildered by it, not grasping his meaning. One day soon afterward, nothing would do but he must be dressed, wheeled out to the pickup, and be loaded in to go there and get his things. Gwen was more willing he go than I thought she'd be, but her reasons were good. First, the old man was insistent about going, and second, it would be good for him to get out of the house anyway, and last, at least he could go and see for himself, and she'd have a few hours' respite.

So off we went, and it was a matter of following the old man's directions, out on the highway, up onto the Parmelee turnoff, until we came to the acreage of a local cattle operation and their feedlot. Elmer told me to turn in the drive, so we did, and I could see he was looking for the house, or trailer, or whatever he had lived in as a young man, for Gwen had told me he'd worked for this same outfit. There was nothing there for him now, of course, so we turned around and headed back toward home, stopping again at the post office in Parmelee to check on the mail. Then we drove home in silence. He never again spoke of having another living space with his complete outfit in it, but it was sad to watch him start to slip away from us.

One thing Gwen told me he'd said sometime the previous year was a reversal of one of his most-repeated instructions: "Don't think about you'self; just think about the people." I've been trying, but it's harder to do than one might suppose. So much over-emphasis on gratifying the self in Western culture, particularly American. But just before the stroke, Gwen had told me he'd said, "Don't think about the people. They been told, and they don't listen. Now they gotta learn their own hard way." She also said that he'd remarked, "The people, they got their own mind." It was plain he was fed up with not being listened to.

Gwen shared some of her other reminiscences with me. Sometimes people would call, former sun dancers, and plead desperately for help with their medical problems, mostly cancer. But in the most recent cases, Elmer was past being able to help, or the person had removed himself or herself from the spirits' aid. "I told 'em not to go 'round to different sun dances," he'd say. That was one lesson I'd learned the hard way, before ever I got to living at Santee. My ex had called in another medicine man from the Twin Cities for a friend who was ill with cancer, who was herself a former sun dancer of Elmer's. I was dragooned into pouring sweat, which I didn't know how to do properly, and helping with the songs at his ceremony, all the while having a terrible feeling about the whole thing. When one does this, seeks help from the spirits of another man's altar when one is already pledged, one loses all help from both. It is offensive to them.

Our marriage fell apart not too long after that, and when I'd given Elmer a rough account of what had happened, early on in my time at Santee, he'd just smiled and said, "I been tellin' the people, but I'm not gon' say one word." And he never did. He really had been an exemplar of the old ways; he was almost never accusatory, unless he was teasing, rarely confrontational, and never rode anybody about anything. On the few occasions when he did get mad at somebody, they really had it coming.

I've already mentioned the evening back in 2001, when one of his boys, Johnson, came over with a bunch of his buddies, drunk, and calling me "Kurt." But, another time, also in 2001, we'd been on a bill-paying/shopping run into Mission, and he'd gone into the Wells Fargo Bank while I waited in the truck. When he came back out a little later, he was grinning. "I had to tell it, that girl in there," he began, and he described a difficulty he'd had with a new girl behind the teller's window. Seems she'd questioned his ID, and he'd gotten impatient. "You musta come down with the rain last night," he repeated, "not to know me."

I seem to recall it was on this same trip in the spring that he told me about Patti's having taken him to the courthouse in Nebraska when she wanted to get married. She went in for a little while, and coming back out to where he was waiting, announced,

"OK, we're married." And he just went along with it for years! But he said to me then, "But I don't think that's right, not unless I said it too."

When I relayed this story to Gwen sometime that summer, she gasped and exclaimed, "You're shittin' me!" He and I had also gone to the tribal legal aid office on the springtime trip, and he mentioned he was getting papers for a legal separation from her. Then he told me about the one-way marriage. Apparently, from what he said, there was no record of marriage to amend. I couldn't believe it myself.

It's not easy to figure why a *wicasa wakan* does the things he does. The spirits could tell him, do this or don't do that, and he'd be under no obligation to explain himself to anyone. Like the time after he'd left Santee, and Patti was insisting by phone that if he came to reclaim his possessions, that he come alone. That was in late summer of 2000. I was there when he was stymied by this, and that time he did explain, "The spirits, what they told me, don't go there; that woman's crazy." That wasn't too hard to figure out!

Meanwhile, back in the summer of 2009, the little Dodge Ram I'd brought the previous year for my fourth year's *wopila* was still sitting in a corner of the yard. I was miffed at Gilli for getting drunk and wrecking it, but I decided to try to get it fixed as a backup vehicle. I went to town a time or two—before I brought the Chev—in the only functioning vehicle they had. It was another pickup, possibly a Ford, and the automatic tranny was shot. Every time you went over fifteen or twenty miles per hour, it went completely out of gear, and you had to coast until it slowed back down before the engine could get any power to the wheels. Horrible! A real blood-pressure raiser.

I had to call a couple of different wrecker services before I found anyone willing to come all the way out to tow it in. Turned out to be the big garage/junkyard on the south of Mission. I paid for the tow and told them to try to get the clutch working again, since that was the main casualty of the crash. It wasn't until after sun dance that we found out that Gilli had hit the post, or tree or whatever, so hard he'd bent the clutch tree, the heavy steel piece that forms the support, and partial housing for the clutch assembly. During that time, I'd made several trips to the NAPA auto parts store in Valentine and a couple visits to the shop to check on the progress. Nothing was getting done. I finally had to take it to another yard, since the owner of the first kept putting me off with delays and absences—mostly to cover the fact that he couldn't fix it himself. At last, it was simply abandoned in a far corner of the second yard as irreparable. Never did go back for it.

Back at the ranch, Sylvan's visits were becoming more and more frequent. He was taking to helping me around Elmer's property and at last made the move from Irene's to the ceremony house. At first, he was helping rebuild the arbor, and during one of the last cool, rainy spells we had, he and I dug a new pit for the outhouse behind the cookshack. It was quite a job and needed two men to get it done in a day. First, we dug a four-foot-square pit down to a depth of five feet or so. We should've made it six, but the rain was really starting to come down, and we still had to lift up the little house, drag it over, and then backfill around the base, plus backfill the old hole. Unfortunately, the wet dirt piled on the tarp was too heavy to move back to the old pit, and we had to wait two days for it to dry.

Once the warm weather had returned, I found myself making quite a few trips to the big junkyard / service shop. First, the problems with Dino's vehicle had returned, and I'd offered to help out. Then Sylvan's little Windstar needed one thing after another.

But we were all more than a little taken aback when he moved his entire family into the ceremony house without so much as a by-your-leave. His wife, granddaughter, and two sons were sleeping there, although the two sons were off working somewhere most of the week. Marie was the wife's name, but the little girl's escapes me. She was a very troubled child, aged six or seven, but was often to be found crawling around on all fours like a much younger child. I made several trips for parts on Sylvan's behalf, and with each one, my motivation changed more from a desire to help out to the realization that as soon as it was running right, he and his could be on their way. There was a debate on in Congress as to whether or not to extend national unemployment benefits, since this was the year that the effects of the big banking houses and the Wall Street speculators, in collusion with the SEC, had finally succeeded in looting the economy to the point of near-total collapse. Now they were running crying to the federals, moaning about how they were too big to fail, and the Bushies couldn't fork it over to them fast enough. Meanwhile, the working unemployed, like Sylvan, had to live hand to mouth for months, waiting fearfully to see if their pittance in benefits would be renewed. Thankfully they were, but we still had them on our hands! To be fair, Sylvan did take over the job of painting the arbor crutches white, and he and Marie even took it upon themselves to paint one of the women's outhouses.

By now, it was early July, and as Elmer had remarked to me years before, in Santee, "Sun dance time gettin' really close now!" But still there was almost no one showing up to help out. Not even Dino, or any of the local sun dancers were stopping by. I recall remarking to Gwen one morning, "You know, Gwen, I kinda hoped that someone in the *tiyospaye* of this man's altar would notice all that I'm trying to do and might give me a name, but there's no *tiyospaye* with this altar." She had to agree, and after all she'd been through on her own, she kinda snorted with laughter at the idea and really busted out when I said, "'Hey, I need help with my vehicle.' That should be my Indian name. That's what they call me."

We'd been having a lot of trouble during all the wet weather the last couple of months with the dirt road to the highway washing out. Several times, the track over the hills was so bad I had to take the Chev onto the grassy margin to get up the last hill. There was too much risk of getting stuck otherwise. But now with the warmer weather, the earth had drained and firmed up, and I finally got around to mowing the parking area north of Elmer's trailer, opposite the cookshack, ceremony house, and arbor. It took all of one afternoon on the new mower since the brush was thick after all the rain. I saw a lot of snakes running for cover as I went through, mostly garters, and once or twice I saw the dark, thick body of a bull snake slipping into a hole.

A few days later, on a grocery / chicken feed / puppy and dog food run into Mission, I stopped at the little deli for another chicken strip basket for Grandpa, and they were out! I'd been making quite a few runs and had bought out their entire supply! "Uh-oh. Grandpa's gonna be mad," I remarked as I picked up my own order (some kind of roast beef and fries combo). Gwen would never eat fast food and rarely let Sage have any, either. In fact, it was only rarely she'd let me pick him up a pack of Slim Jims or jerky.

Sage and I had gone into Mission the weekend before the Fourth of July, and we'd picked up a modest supply of fireworks. Sage had some crackers and roman candles and the like, whilst I contented myself with a few fountains and a rocket or two. For once, with all the wet weather, there was little danger of sparking off a prairie fire. We had a good time setting them off on the holiday weekend.

I had not given up on my intention of going up on the hill for *hanblechiya* that year, and when time permitted, I'd work on my flags and ties. Just as in the previous year, however, not only was I busy helping run the outfit, but there were interruptions every time I sat down to work on the flags and ties. Sometimes it would be Gwen on the CB. I'd set up a home station in the kitchen and, with the help of a borrowed antenna I found in the toolshed, installed a little mobile unit in the van. This was in case of some emergency, in case she needed me in a hurry.

I'd also followed her suggestion to pick up a baby monitor, with the mike in Elmer's bedroom. That way if Gilli or one of his kids snuck in the back way and started hassling him, we'd know about it. At least Gwen might. She had more Lakota than I did and could pick up a few phrases. As it turned out, Gilli did show up a time or two, but the conversations were always in Lakota, and we had to try to piece together what was said by Elmer's reaction. Seems like one time he got the old man agitated by telling him he was going to run Irene off, get her back up to White River, and get Elmer back onto his old property. Of course, this never happened. Then there was the business with Norman and Shannon, how they'd taken the titles to all of Grandpa's vehicles, plus god knows what other paperwork, including that of the vehicle he'd given to Gwen. We found out later he was photocopying them and forging his own name! Gwen told me that Elmer had once said to her, "Norman's gon' try and steal the sun dance." Then there were the phone calls, at any and all hours, from Johnson's wife, demanding to know if he was there and never believing us when we said he wasn't. Sometimes she'd put their young daughter on: "Is my daddy there?" she'd ask. Hassles from Elmer's relatives were all but unceasing that whole spring and summer. I can't recall them all, but if I were to, this would be a far longer book!

After many visits to the shop, Sylvan's vehicle was at last ready to roll. Things were getting tense, at least as far as I was concerned. The most recent interruption in my getting my flags and ties ready for *hanblechiya* had been when he had shown up directly beneath my camper's window after returning from a meeting over to Crow Dog's. He'd been given a commemorative

Tshirt that he presented to me as a token of esteem for all I'd
done. I accepted it and shook hands, but it was at least two sizes
too small. Then we had to go on our last trip to the shop—to
get his vehicle and pay for the repairs. He brought along Marie
and the grandchild, and while we were there, waiting for it to be
brought up, I spotted a jack lying next to the vehicle it had once
belonged to. I picked it up, went into the shop, and paid for it,
along with the repair bill. But on our way back to his van, Sylvan
noticed another Windstar that was the same as his vehicle. He
pulled a reservoir tank out of it, stuffed it up under his shirt, and
we drove off without his paying for it! On the way back, Marie
had a fit of the nervous giggles, saying, "Grandpa stole that white
plastic thing!" I just thought it was a bad example.

It was about this time too, when, early one morning, I was
trying to sneak in a little work on the ties and flags before beginning work, and who should come right over the hill and into the
ceremony house but Johnson. He was the one of Elmer's boys
we'd had the most trouble from, after Gilli. He was the one I'd
had to dump off, drunk, at his girlfriend's place back in the
spring of 2001. He'd shown up drunk more than once while I
was there this year too but never admitted to it: "I'm not drunk.
I'm hungover." It was getting so the tribal police wouldn't even
respond to our calls anymore, we'd had to call so often.

Anyhow, both of Sylvan's grown boys were in there this
morning when in barged Johnson, with his big walking stick,
and tried to give them the bum's rush. I found out about the hul-
laballoo a few moments later when Lala started barking. Sylvan
came out back where my van was parked, followed by Johnson
and Lala. Johnson wasn't drunk, for a change, but he did sound
like he had a few in him. Sylvan said something about his trying to throw them out, and Johnson started defending himself. I
lost it and lit into him, yelling that he had no business trying to
run anyone off when we'd had to run him so often, and so on.

That was all the cue Lala needed. He was standing right next to Johnson and totally had my back; he just reached up and bit him on the hand, fast but not too hard, and he felt it. That was all it took. He shut up and backed down and sort of wandered back to Irene's.

Sylvan was kind of mad and told me Johnson was lucky his boys knew they were guests, or they might have given him a good seeing-to. Well, there was no way I could go back to making prayer ties and the flags after that—too angry, too much adrenaline in the system. So, I went back into the mobile home and, over a cup of coffee, told Gwen what had just happened. She asked me if I knew why Johnson carried that stick all the time. "It's for snakes," she said. "He's afraid of snakes, so he always carries that." She went on to say how she'd once read him the riot act when he'd come over drunk. She'd told him how his family missed him and how he was letting his dad down with his drunken ways. She said he broke down and started crying, but nothing changed.

"Well, keep it up," I said. "It may not do any good, but it can't hurt."

Since it was getting so close to sun dance, the window on going up on the hill was starting to close. I was nowhere near done with what I needed to finish—mostly due to the interruptions by the relatives and Sylvan. Every time I paid for a repair on his vehicle, I hoped it would be the last, but it never was. Inevitably, something else would go. I don't want to give the impression that Sylvan and Marie were no-account: Whenever I'd have to go into the ceremony house while they were there, Marie would rush around and hand me a cup of coffee and a nice piece of fry bread. When I mentioned it to Gwen, she responded, "That's really traditional."

But I have to back up a bit again and tell about the pipe carving. A few weeks prior to the confrontation with Johnson, Gwen and I were talking about the pipe. I remembered a pipe Elmer had carved back in 2000. It was a smaller one with an orange-colored layer running through it, and he had carved little spiders running around the bowl. He always gave them away, and at that time, I had a neighbor in the little Nebraska town I was living in who remarked that he always wanted an Indian pipe for his collection. I recall I even brought him up for monthly ceremony once at the new place in Santee. Well, I told Elmer he'd been a pretty good neighbor to me and asked him for the spider pipe. He almost didn't get it, it was so nice, but he did. Turns out, he wasn't worthy to keep a *canunpa*, let alone pray with one. At first, I couldn't understand why he fell down and injured his foot severely within a few months of having gotten it—but the next year he was arrested and eventually went to prison for tampering with his niece and granddaughter. Tore that family right up; I shoulda kept it, then I'd at least have a pipe made by Grandpa.

I mentioned some of this, at least about that pipe, to Gwen, and she said she'd been wanting an eagle pipe herself. So I went into the old trading post in Mission, and the fellow there had one slab of stone big enough for two pipes. Since Sylvan had been doing so much nice artwork, I approached him about carving a set of pipes for us. He said sure, he could do it.

Next, I went to the local NAPA auto parts store and bought Elmer a floor jack for working on vehicles. He'd had one, years before, but like so many of his things, it had been stolen. That's what he told me when I brought it in to show to him: "I useta have one o' them, but somebody stole it." I'd noticed a fancy-twist pipe stem in one of his drawers once when we couldn't find where he'd hidden the keys to the Chevy and he couldn't remember where he'd put them. Anyway, I offered to trade him the jack for the pipe stem, and he agreed. When I mentioned this to Gwen and gave the stem to her for her pipe, Gorgie was present. She asked me, "Karl, did you ever see a movie called

Thunderheart?" I knew what she meant: the trading scene with
Grandpa Albert White Hat, in which he trades a rock to Val
Kilmer's character for a pair of Ray-Bans, and Graham Greene
ends up with them.

So I got the stone and some files and tools over to Sylvan and
asked him to do it in a good way. He set to work. All I needed
then was a stem for my pipe, which was to be a spider pipe, for
him to carve it to. Soon afterward, I happened to be at the Starlite
store on the west end of Mission, and a pipe stem was lying on
the counter when I walked in. The lady running the place that
day said, "I don't know where that came from or how it got
there!" It wasn't priced, even, so I offered her a fair one, and she
agreed. Funny how things can happen when you're around a
medicine man.

Sylvan had another occupation, for which I'd offered him
a good wage for his time. Meanwhile, while not taking care of
Elmer, Gwen was busy in the garden and working on her camper.

With the weather now warm and fair, it was the perfect time
to fix her camper's leaky roof. I'd had to go to the lumberyard
in Valentine for a gallon of silicone roof sealant. It didn't take
Sage and me long to give it a good thick coat once we'd gotten
the ladder in place, and we soon had the gallon used up. Gwen
was trying also to coax a little effort out of Sylvan and Marie's
granddaughter. There was a stack of five-gallon plastic buckets
she was going to use for food storage, and she tried to get the
little girl to clean them out. She had brushes and the hose, but
it was no use. As soon as Gwen left to light a cigarette for Elmer,
the little one just wandered off. I had to warn her repeatedly to
stay out of the chicken yard and coop. She'd get in there and
chase the birds around, which is no good for egg laying. The most
disturbing thing, though, was what she thought was fun. A pair
of swifts of some kind had built their nest right above the door to
the cookshack. Whenever anyone came close, they'd take off and

fly around the area very fast, but low to the ground. This poor little girl would take a big kitchen knife in her hand and chase the birds around with it. Creepiest thing I ever saw, her laughing as she did that. Her grandpa Sylvan caught her at it once while he was walking by and hollered at her to stop. She did, and there was no chance she'd ever even get close to catching one, but it was still a bad thing to have seen.

The wind began to set in from the west in the afternoons more and more every day. The crutches in the sun-dance arbor were all painted now, but with all the moisture in the earth, the whole grounds would have to be mowed at least once more before sun dance. So I was painting the outhouses in the colors we had—one mostly yellow with a red design, one mostly red with some black, and blue and green for the main one behind the cookshack, and blue and red and black with a design for another. I can't recall what we painted on the ladies' one down by the dance arbor.

One morning the wind had been blowing strongly for two or three days, making doing anything almost impossible. I was up early as usual, and I fed the dogs after having my coffee in my camper. I got it in my head to walk along the front, or south, side of the ceremony house / cookshack. As I reached the south end, I saw it: a big yellow-tailed hawk's wing feather lying in the grass and twitching to every gust. I put down a little tobacco and said a prayer of thanks. I kept walking, though, and soon found another—a much smaller feather, but obviously from the same bird. I immediately went back into the mobile home, where Gwen was in the back room taking care of Elmer. The coffee was already on, so I got a cup and sat down, with the feathers on the table before me. Gwen breezed past them at first, talking about how Grandpa was doing, so after a bit I sort of pointed them out to her. (All the Indians just laugh when I try to point with lips.)

"Where did you find them?" she asked.

"Just past the ceremony house," I replied.

"Karl, that's ... You know how the wind's been blowing here!"

"Yeah, I know. I guess somebody thinks I've been doing a good job here." I gave Gwen the little feather and put the big one inside a flat plastic bag with a little sage. Then I tacked it up inside the van for a blessing.

And now at last, with only a week or so to go before sun dance, here comes Dino. I hadn't been there for the sweat before Grandpa's last ceremony, after which Elmer had complained to her that Dino had put on too many rocks, soon after which he suffered his second stroke. But hearing her speak of it, I realized he'd told her himself. She had been with him for months on end, just about as long as I'd been in Santee, and I knew that after a while the old man would open up if he thought he could trust you.

Around this time too, but before the big wind, Gwen said he'd told her about the big snake. The floor in the hallway between the bathroom and Elmer's bedroom was pretty weak in spots. In one place it had given way entirely, and Gwen said that Grandpa had told her that a big bull snake had been coming in there for a while at night and visiting with the old medicine man. Now I recall, he'd told this to me too. I didn't know what to make of it, but I believed him, for I'd never known him to lie about anything. *Anything.* And I'd seen big snakes in the area. It reminded me of a time earlier in the year, also during a period of stormy weather. One of the Eagle dancers, Sonny, had been there for a little time, and there was a big tornado-producing storm coming in. Gwen told me she'd gone back to ask Grandpa what they should do about it, and he said, "It's all right. I got my *canunpa* out. It's gon' go around us." And it did. Twisters around Mission and Parmelee, but not where we were, in between.

So, anyway, Dino comes out at last, with an uncle of his and one of his adopted boys, and bringing back Vern Yellowhawk! Gwen and I had printed up and posted a set of rules by the front door, mostly about no drugs, alcohol, firearms, or cameras were allowed. One of the first things Vern did was come up to the front door and read them, and I went out there and wedged myself in between him and the doorway. Gwen was mightily pissed off at his being there, and I wasn't any too pleased myself. This was Dino flagrantly going against what the old man wanted. The medicine man who was the reason for all of us being there had said he didn't want this guy around, and if Dino had been present and helping out like he should have been, he'd have known it. But that might not have made any difference.

Anyway, Dino comes in, and we started having sweats again. Gwen was sticking close to the mobile home, since she didn't trust Vern being around. I was beginning the final mowing and still helping Sylvan with the last few repairs on his vehicle. At last, however, he said it was ready. He managed to finish his work on the two *canunpas* around the same time. I'd bought some red felt, and Gwen had gotten on her computer and looked up the inventory on the website for Dakota Drum in Rapid City. We looked over the fantastic selection of Indian-made pipe bags, since it is important to honor the pipe as soon as it's ready by having the red felt and sage to wrap it in and a nicely decorated pipe bag to carry it in. The sage was no problem! We each picked out a good-looking bag and sent in the order. Gwen knew the lady who owns and runs the store, and she confirmed that they were on their way.

By now, it was mid-July, and we were getting more and more phone traffic from people who wanted to check on the first day of purification. It was the same time as always, the first weekend in August. The weather was getting downright hot by now, so much so that Elmer's bedroom at the west end of the trailer was all but intolerable in the afternoons. So it was down to Valentine for me, to pick up a window air conditioner at the hardware store. When I got back, Sylvan and I rigged up a support stand of scrap lumber and got it fixed in the old man's north window. It was good to have another pair of hands on call, but Elmer was starting to get agitated about "them Indians in the ceremony house."

I had to start dropping a few hints to Sylvan about how, with sun dance coming up, there were going to be people needing to use the space. His two boys had gone back to Gordon, but now another child of his, or Marie's—someone's teenage daughter—was in there with them, and it was all getting to be a bit much. Sometimes Sylvan would take off in a vehicle we knew nothing about, driven by a friend or relative, and be gone for hours without telling us, and there went the extra pair of hands. We found out later that Dino was recruiting him into his little band of followers and getting other sun dancers involved in his machinations.

Bedbugs and New Furniture

EVERY SO OFTEN, I'D HAVE TO TAKE THE CHEV INTO MISSION to gas up and fill the cans for the mowers. Sylvan and Elmer came along on one of these trips, and we didn't go for just a fill-up. The bedbugs had gotten so bad, I'd decided to call in a fumigator. Before this, indeed over the preceding month or more, Gwen had gone to town on the inside of the trailer. She stripped off everything from the kitchen shelves and walls, repainted the whole room very nicely, and put up some new sets of blinds. This was when she'd told me of the roach invasion of the previous winter. It seems they'd invaded the whole kitchen, shelves, drawers, and all. They'd even gotten as far back as Elmer's bedroom before she'd gotten them all killed off. In telling me, she said that when she'd mentioned it to Gorgie, she'd said, "An infestation? You know what that means, don't you? It means someone's praying some bad medicine on you." From her description of it, there may have been something to this. I completely believed Elmer's story of how a jealous dance rival had shot some bad medicine into his knee, and this seemed akin to that. Both were consistent with what I've heard some bad medicine people can do, if they use the power in the wrong way.

So the young man who was the exterminator came up, just when the company I'd called said he would. Very polite, told us we'd have to stay out until at least four o'clock to let the stuff die down. He also asked me if we were a family. I had to say no, that I was just a friend helping out. It had started to feel like a family, though, at least to me—Gwen, me, Sage, and Grandpa, plus the dogs and cat. One night, the three of us had sat down to supper around the kitchen table, and something just clicked. Felt like a dad settin' down. Pretty good feeling, although Sage was never my boy, or Gwen my woman. I guess the unconscious mind makes fairly simple assumptions, given the right situation, and makes you feel like maybe there's more going on than actually is.

Anyway, Sylvan, Grandpa, and I had gone into Mission, leaving Gwen and Sage to hang out at the ceremony house with Marie and the kids. Elmer had pretended (?) to be pretty cantankerous with the exterminator fella, raising his fist when told he'd have to stay away from his home, just playin'. The young man took it well, saying he would cry if Grandpa hit him. I had mentioned to Gorgie during one of her recent visits that I'd broken down and gone in to White Horse Trading Post to get some flute CDs that no one else had. She'd answered, "Yeah, don't you hate it when you do that?" The Englishwoman who ran the place was a pothead, for one thing; I'd smelled it on her sweater.

I also knew she and her husband, a Lakota, had set up their own ceremony house and were copying from Elmer. "Monkey see, monkey do; that's the way the monkey learns," Grandpa had remarked to me the night back in 2000 when we'd been discussing them. I'd seen her singing ceremony songs with a glass of wine in her hand, and she wore a ring with a pentagram on it, which convinced Elmer beyond doubt she was a witch.

At any rate, the three of us were in Mission, it was a bright, sunny day, and there was a roadside vendor set up in an empty lot next to the church, which was across an alley from the trading post. I pulled off the road, and the first thing Elmer said was, "You goin' to church?"

I said, "Hell, no!"

We got out and inspected this guy's goods. He had what might have been the contents of a powwow vendor's booth on a flatbed trailer, to which he'd added some shelving. There was an upright rack of earrings, some turkey-feather fans, rolls of artificial sinew, and beaded key rings, among the rest. At his request, I bought a pair of earrings for Sylvan to give to Marie. I got a key chain for Gwen. We'd recently changed the locks on the mobile home and the ceremony house, so I thought it'd come in handy. Unfortunately, that turned into another worry. Once we found out Sylvan was being recruited by Dino, that key could have easily been duplicated and fallen into who knows whose hands. We'd had to have given him a copy, obviously.

Well, we passed the time there in town, I bought some more gas, got us all some lunch at the inevitable deli with the chicken-strip basket, and last, I went in to White Horse. I picked up a few more flute CDs and chatted a bit with Alva, the proprietress. The subject got onto Elmer, since she remembered me from previous visits and pretty much knew why I'd be back in the area. I told her about the stroke he'd suffered, but not too much about recent events, figuring it wasn't her business. But she got to asking questions more closely and asked me if the old man was around. I had to admit he was right outside in the pickup, and nothing would do, but she must go out to say hello and shake Grandpa's hand. When I got back to the vehicle, I was apprehensive, and the old man was mad about it.

"That white woman's a witch," he grumbled at me. We picked Sylvan up from whatever he'd gone off about after lunch and headed home.

When we got back, there was still a little less than two hours to go before we could safely reenter the trailer. Elmer was sitting in his foldable wheelchair in the shade of the ceremony house, and some of us were sitting at the picnic tables in front of the cookshack. Elmer began insisting he wanted to go back inside, and after a little while of arguing back and forth, we finally did. I was concerned about the toxicity, but he needed to relieve himself, which he couldn't do alone.

That's still embarrassing for me to recall, being so dense as not to get right away why he wanted back in, but there was one more bright moment: I'd overshot the turnoff to his place, after the turn off the highway. He'd turned and asked me, "You goin' back to Mission? Hah?"

"No, Grandpa. I just missed the turn."

And, at last, the place was free of those damned bedbugs!

That was a Friday, if I remember right. The next Monday, Sylvan and Marie were out painting outhouses, and I was trying to get my bills paid. I had a notebook with the phone numbers and some of the account numbers and addresses of the various utility companies. I'd been away two months now, and I just managed to get a good roaming signal on my cell phone. I had to sit in my camper with that little radio transmitter right up against my ear and make call after call, sit through the interminable prompts and menus, and write down the amounts and addresses where I needed to send them. After ten or fifteen minutes, I noticed an unpleasant burning sensation just behind my right ear, which is where I was holding the phone. I gave it a rest for a bit but had to get it finished, because being so much farther west meant a day or two postal-delivery time. By the time I was done, my ear felt like it was on fire. I put the cell phone away and have scarcely used it since. But by Tuesday, my head was hurting so badly, I had to go to the emergency room. Ordinarily, I'd have probably gotten some over-the-counter eardrops, made flags and ties, and loaded my *canunpa* for a doctoring ceremony, but, sadly, that was no longer an option.

The rez emergency room was about as grim a place as I've ever seen the inside of. Through the open door to the next room, I could hear a police officer and an intern going over the catalogue of injuries sustained by a Lakota woman who'd been battered by her husband or boyfriend. Then the doc came in, looked in my ear, and asked me, "Have you been swimming? Looks like you've got an ear infection."

"No, like I said. I've just had to use my cell phone for an extended period."

Apparently, I'd suffered a radio burn, internally. Radiant power, whether it's radiation, microwaves, or plain radio signals, is still power, and all the stories I've heard about those little devices everyone thinks are so wonderful causing brain tumors, I believe 'em. I've been on anti-inflammatories and steroidal ear drops, and that damned burn is still giving me problems to this day! Like I really needed a complication with my sinuses! Thank you, Motorola. Don't call me; I won't call you.

I need to recall one happy occurrence, however, lest it be overshadowed. It was early in the summer one morning, and I was backing up the Chev to the ramp, where Gwen was waiting with Grandpa in his wheelchair on the back porch, for our first trip to Mission. I got out and opened the passenger door for Elmer, after having opened the tailgate for stowing the chair. As Gwen was getting him down the ramp, he turned and spoke to her. I couldn't catch what was said at first, but the next moment, they were closer, and I heard him tell her, "He's got porcupine medicine." Meaning, of course, that I smelled bad, but also that he'd finally remembered me from our time at Santee!

Gwen replied, "Oh, Grandpa, you're too funny!" And we loaded him in and were off. That was close to the best time I had at Rosebud that summer.

I wish I could recall more of what he said as we went along. I remember lighting his smokes for him and how fastidious he still was, brushing the last speck of ash off his black jeans until they were clean. He'd recovered enough to fumble one out of the pack on his own, but he could barely get it to his lips, and flicking the spark wheel on a Bic was just out of reach. I was pretty tickled at his recollection—but like most good things that summer, it didn't last long.

Speaking of lighters, one odd thing that happened was his difficulty in getting lighters to work at all. It happened that a green Bic I'd gotten for him just quit. I'd never known one to just quit when there was still fuel inside, and it was still sparking, but this one did. He hollered up to us one afternoon, while I was inside during the hottest part of the day, "Take it 'way; this goddamn lighter's no good!" Sure enough, it wouldn't light. So after a tobacco run across the line into Valentine, I found him one I knew he'd like. Bic came out that year with a line of animal-themed lighters: There were a buck, a bear, an eagle, and one with a black widow spider. I bought the last two they had. This happened after the green lighter's nonperformance had been repeated by at least two others. When I got back, I gave the eagle lighter to Gwen and then went on back to the old man's bedroom. "Grandpa, I got you a lighter for that old one that wouldn't work." He took it and held it up close. "Iktomi," he whispered and shook my hand. That one worked for him.

While Elmer and I were away on one or the other of our trips to Mission, Gwen was never idle. The relatives who'd been taking credit for taking care of him over the short period during the winter when she was at Nico's were unable or simply unwilling to do the work of caring for an elder who was, after his stroke, incontinent. Gwen had told me the Gilli had been one of the last to leave and that she found Elmer lying in his bed, caked in about three days' worth of his own filth. So the mattress and carpet were in a bad way. I'd made several runs to Mission and even Valentine before I'd found the correct Febreze product she'd asked me to get. Once I had, though, she went to town, washed everything that'd fit inside the washer, and soaked everything else with the stuff, to get the bedroom livable again. The little double-wide was in ten times better shape than it had been in late May.

On another trip to Valentine, I'd become friendly with the couple who ran the consignment store where I'd found the new kitchen chairs. The gentleman showed me around their warehouse, and I was able to get a deal on some new furniture for the living room. The old couch was falling apart, and all the cushions and pillows now had dead bedbugs in 'em. Ick. But with all this traveling, it was getting harder to get the keys away from Grandpa. I had to ask him twice or three times a week, and although he never bitched me out again after I'd handed him some backtalk that one time, he still made it difficult. He demanded it be brought right back, and with Gilli's visits getting more frequent as sun-dance time approached, he'd taken to hiding them in his shorts. Eeeeww! "Grandpa, that's nasty!" Gwen exclaimed once.

As to Gilli's visits, they were surreptitious. We sometimes didn't know he was back there until we heard raised voices in Lakota, and it became apparent he was winding up the old man for his own benefit. There was no sign of Irene and her bunch leaving the old homestead up on Ironwood, but Gilli was worming his way back into the old man's affairs. I'll never forget the time when he went and picked up Elmer's lunch at the Elderly Assistance office and kept it for himself. This, after one morning's visit when he'd come in the front door all aboveboard, insisting on shaking hands, and when he left, I kept on wiping my palm off on my pants leg as soon as he was out the door. We were still getting some calls from sun dancers whose names were on the list he'd stolen the year before about when sun dance was going to be.

Now the nights were quite short, and the weather was hot. Late July in South Dakota. The winds would mostly get up around noon, out of the west, and sweep across the endless prairie all the way from the Rockies. They were becoming unusually strong too, as they had been last year. The mornings were still cool, though, and peaceful early on. I'd get up early, have coffee, greet and feed the dogs, and usually start my day in the toolshed/ shop, trying to keep Elmer's machines in order. I was minding what had been said about getting the place looking good for the old man's funeral and trying to keep the tall weeds and grasses down along the margins and around the arbor. Immense blue sky overhead, gentle breeze in the morning, and quiet. We were several miles from the road leading to the main highway, with hills between, so it was just silent, as nature combines silence out of a thousand natural sounds.

But I need to backtrack just a week or two and tell of a morning when I was headed east on the highway out of Elmer's, toward the old Rosebud Agency. I was on the big hill, past Crow Dog's Paradise, on the long downslope that leads into the town itself, when I passed an Indian couple pulled over onto the shoulder. The lady was sitting inside, but as I passed the man, who was standing at the rear of the vehicle, he watched me go by with a sort of an almost pleading look. I can't recall what it was I was headed in for, but I pulled around and headed back. Turned out, they'd simply run out of gas a mile or three short of the closest convenience store. After I got out of the Chev and walked over, the man (whose name was Leadercharge) told me that a carful of younger people had stopped, and he'd given them his gas can and a few dollars and that they'd simply run off with it.

This had been an hour or so before I drove by. "These people!" he exclaimed as I drove him into the agency. I think he may have said his first name was Doug. Somehow, from the moment I saw him standing there, the whole event seemed charged with significance. Like this was something for me to do, and it was important that I do it. Sometimes even a *wasicu* can feel it, when the grandfathers are watching. I paid for his gas—may have bought him a small replacement can, I don't remember—and took them back to their vehicle. Had to do it like that too; leaving a vehicle unattended on those rez back roads is an invitation to vandalism. I went back to whatever errand I'd been on, finished it, and went back to Grandpa's. But that was the same day Dino brought me my feather.

By now, Sylvan had finished the pipes for Gwen and me. I'd taken the flat stem I'd gotten at Starlite and, using my butane lighter and a nail, had burned a random series of dots onto it, to represent hailstones. Then I'd sent it to Sylvan. I'd gotten some red felt for him to wrap them in, and he brought them over to the mobile home very happily one morning. We all went into the living room to look them over, and his granddaughter perched herself on the couch right next to where they were lying on the coffee table. The neglect really showed on that kid. She did some-thing so wrong, especially for an NDN girl, just for the attention: swinging her leg right alongside the pipe that was to be for me, within a hair of kicking it off the table. I finally had to tell her to cut it out. The stems fit, at least they seemed to at first, so I paid Sylvan off. It was quite a fair price, but what he said next was a revelation: "It's the first time I've ever done this!" Not what he'd said before!

So with the felt and the pipe bags we'd gotten from Dakota Drum, we were all set. Sylvan was happy about being paid and mentioned that before the pipes were used, they should be blessed in ceremony. But when I asked Gwen about it, she said they were sacred from the moment they were finished and the stem was first fitted on. I was beginning to go to her more and more for advice on such matters, since if what she'd told me was true, she'd been around the people and their ways for some ten years and had the respect of the grandmothers at Pine Ridge for having served the people. She told me that Sage's father, one of Crow Dog's boys who was a pipe carver himself, had told her that. Ordinarily, I would have taken a question like that right to Elmer, but he was getting harder and harder to reach. He was spending more and more time in the world of his own past; he thought he was back in Ironwood and working for that cattle outfit in Parmelee.

When he was fully with us, he was often frustrated and angry at being so dependent on others. Once, soon after the pipes were done, he called me back into his bedroom and told me to get some electrical wire and run it from the outlet in the wall to just over his bed. The reason he wanted it was pretty obvious, and I refused to do it—it was maybe the first time I'd ever told him no about anything he'd asked me for.

By now, some of the old-time sun dancers were beginning to arrive: Jason from Lincoln; Alan, whom I'd known from Santee; some of the local people from Rosebud; and some of the new folks. Lehr had been in touch with Gorgie, or had called Gwen, and said he wouldn't be able to make it this year, which disappointed me. I'd been looking forward to seeing him again. In fact, I was getting so burned out from all of Gilli's and the relatives' nonsense and Sylvan's unending need for funds for his car that I was considering bugging out myself.

However, before I get into the last week before sun dance and the beginning of purification, a few more incidents from the time just prior. The winds were getting so strong during the latter part of July that tornadoes were forming and sometimes touching down at points west, north, and even east of Ironwood and Parmelee. We were keeping tabs on the TV and radio weather reports, and one evening in particular was very threatening. I told Gwen that I'd learned a prayer tie from Grandma Darlene about that: Make one full-sized white flag, leave a length of string on both ends, tie six white ones on one side, and use the other length to secure it all to the west side of the dwelling. She agreed that it would probably be a good idea, so I did.

By this time, Sylvan and his family were out of the ceremony house. We'd had a confrontation. I'd hitched up his vehicle to the Chev and towed it over to the shop for its final repair. He drove it once, then had to have it towed back by a relative who was on the tribal police force. When I saw it was back in a non-running capacity, I just went ballistic. Started yelling at him while the officer-cousin just stood there and grinned. Can't recall a word I said. But the gist of it was: I wasn't paying for any more repairs, and he needed to get himself and his family out of there because sun dance was starting soon. I was too angry then to remember now how that scene ended, but all the Windstar needed was a simple part installed, and the ceremony house was vacated soon thereafter. His family went back to Gordon, but Sylvan ended up staying locally elsewhere. But by now, he was firmly embroiled with Dino's faction, which would come up later.

To get back to it, on the evening of the tornado, Gwen and Sage were getting pretty nervous about the storm. They had their bugout bags by the front door, and Gwen asked me repeatedly if I didn't think we should get Grandpa into his wheelchair and over to the (now-empty) ceremony house. I said I thought not, since I'd already put up the white flag and ties just outside Grandpa's bedroom, and I didn't think the thunder beings would hit a home occupied by a *wicasa wakan*. What I didn't say was that both the mobile home and the ceremony house were of fairly flimsy construction, and neither would offer anything in the way of shelter if we were in the direct path of a twister. The situation put me in mind of something that had happened years earlier in Santee.

There had been a story in the news about another reservation, in North Dakota, that had been hit by a tornado, and Patti had remarked on how unusual that was. Elmer had just grinned and said, "They got no medicine man up there." There aren't too many of the real ones left, but the ones who are have talked about how hard it makes it to hold back what's coming, with their numbers dwindling.

Anyway, we stayed with Grandpa in the mobile home, and the storm passed us by—barely. For a moment, I thought it was all over. The wind was so loud it had almost that freight-train sound one hears of. The gusts were shaking the little trailer, coming closer and closer together. Finally, we heard it was sighted just to the north of Parmelee, which was north of us, heading east. However, the last gust raced along the north side of the mobile home with an impact you could feel through the walls. As if a giant had run his hand all down that side.

Before I bring this narrative back to its present, I want to do a page for Sage. The previous year, some of the sun dancers had brought him a new bike, plus other toys appropriate for a boy his age. But even so, it was kinda hard on him out there. With his mom having to devote so much of her time to Elmer's care, he was forever getting himself into trouble by getting on her computer, playing games, and not deleting them when he was done. I was utterly unfamiliar with computers and their uses then, less so now, but anyone could see it upset her. But it was hard to blame him much. There was no one within miles his own age for him to play with, so he was very into his job of feeding the chickens and collecting their eggs every day. He also had great fun playing with the puppies, who were both getting a lot bigger now. They were out of the roly-poly stage and getting to look like dogs.

Sage was incredibly polite and well-spoken for a ten-year-old. He was always willing when asked to do any chore. I tried to get him in the habit of always carrying around a plastic baggie around with him, as I did, to take care of any dog poop wherever he found it. I was a little too hard on him about it once. Gwen

had to come to his defense and point out that the pair of shorts
he had on had no pockets. Also, one time the female puppy had
gotten tangled underneath the front porch, and I was urging him
to get down there and get her loose. He was having some trouble
with it, and when I got him to go back in a second time, he saw
a dead mouse and pulled back, exclaiming, "I don't wanna get
sick!" I tried to get him to free the animal himself, but he finally
refused to go back in, and I had to get her free. I could tell he was
mad at me. The next day I apologized for being so insistent, and
he was cool about it: "That's OK!" But I suspect I shouldn't have
backed down.

Then there was the time Johnson came over drunk and
wouldn't leave. While I was outside on the porch, keeping him
from entering and telling him he had to leave, Sage was running
around the yard in front of us, grinning like a monkey, obviously
delighted with the situation for some reason. I finally told him,
"Sage, go inside and tell your ma to call the police."

He said, "OK!" and darted right inside.

That made Johnson get up and lurch off in the direction of
Irene's. That was a help.

But just before the other sun dancers began to arrive, Elmer
and I had taken another, longer trip to Valentine to get the old
man some air and give Gwen a chance to move the new furniture
around. It was getting so that, whenever someone would drop by
for a visit, they'd actually look a little shocked to see how nice
the place was getting to be. I'd helped to clean off the big mirror
in the hall, which had had to be covered many times—whenever
we'd had to do ceremony in the trailer before the ceremony house
was built. Gwen had asked me to get new blinds for the windows,
and she'd made some new curtains, so it really was looking nice.
I was feeling like the man of the house too, since it was my job to
carry out the garbage to the Dumpster.

So Elmer and I set off for Valentine. It was still cooler in the mornings, and for once, it wasn't too windy. I'd never seen Rosebud and the prairie looking so green, after all the rain. We got sort of a late start, so we stopped in Mission for lunch, right outside the little deli where I'd get him his chicken-strip baskets and the usual sandwich and fries for myself. We ate together in the pickup, so feeding him wasn't a problem. One had to hold a drink with a straw for him to sip on and make sure the bites he took weren't too large. He'd developed a tendency to gobble his food, as I'd found out once, having left him to eat by himself one afternoon. I'd gone to eat my own lunch in the living room. He'd told me, when I'd placed his food on his tray, "When I eat, I like to really eat!" But after a moment or two away, I heard him start choking, just as Gwen had warned me he might, and I stood by kinda helpless while he fought to get it down and start breathing again! When he did, he gave me kind of an accusing look, accompanied by a garbled exclamation I couldn't quite understand. But it sounded like a protest against the unfairness of not being able to even simply eat on his own.

Back in Mission on our way to Valentine, I'd made the mistake of chatting in the deli with a Lakota woman who was very rumpled looking. When she claimed to be a relative of Elmer's, I told her he was sitting in the pickup right outside. Big mistake. What does she do but lean in the window and start begging him for money! I felt like such a dunce. I should have seen it coming. Elmer just gave her a dollar, shook her hand, and luckily didn't make the connection between her and myself.

Well, we had a nice, long drive down to Valentine, where I was to pick up some more smokes for everybody. But Elmer had to relieve himself, so it was out with the wheelchair in the parking lot of the big convenience store / gas station on the highway. Always a lot of traffic there, and as I got him settled in, a fellow came up to us, a white man in motorcycle leathers who asked me if I needed any help. I did. Elmer, slight as he was, wasn't easy to maneuver into his chair. I don't know how Gwen had been able to do it by herself all those months. I was grateful for his assistance and told him so. The man shook hands with Elmer and asked if he was a full-blood Indian. I said he was and that he was one of the last of the old-time Sioux medicine men. Elmer assumed a look of great dignity, and this man said he was personally glad that his people had whipped Custer. Elmer smiled handsomely and just nodded, shaking his hand right back.

After I'd gotten Elmer taken care of and filled up the Chev and parked him in the shade, I had to go back in and use the facilities myself. The most bizarre thing happened. There were several other men in there, and I was a little stressed out by now. Not just the wheelchair business, but all of it—Sylvan and his family and his vehicle, the relatives, especially Gilli, and especially Norman, and especially Johnson, and Dino bringing Vern back around. It was all beginning to tell. So this grinning, loud-talking white guy comes charging into the wash-up area of the rest room. He zeroes in on me for some reason and is spouting some gibberish about needing to take a leak and how it's harder for guys who are well hung, know what I mean? I quietly responded, "I don't care to discuss it."

And he won't take the hint, but gets right up in my grille and says, "What?"

And I let him have it! *"I Don't Care To Discuss It Any Further!"* Sucked all the air outta the men's room, I did. No one could say a thing, including Mr. Anatomy.

I've never had the karmic sendings come in such close balance before or since, first one out of the light, then one from the darker places. So I got the smokes, and we headed back to Elmer's.

Another thing coming to a head around this time concerned the issues we were having with Lorna. Another of Elmer's old-timers, she lived locally and was, with Gorgie, responsible for helping to manage the account holding Grandpa's funds, which had been sent and donated by various dancers and supporters. She'd helped out the year before, but I had hardly seen her around in the time I'd been there this year. Gwen was kinda down on her, and beyond the usual business of a woman being territorial about her home in general and kitchen in particular, I have to say she had some right. I noticed once when Lorna came in how she just threw her keys on the kitchen counter. Didn't say hello or offer to shake hands with Gwen or myself and just rushed back to talk to Elmer.

Gwen and Sage had both warned me against eating any of the food Lorna would bring over. "She goes to all the wakes for people," Gwen said, "and takes some of the food and leaves it in her car for a couple of days. Then she comes out here and gives it to Grandpa. It makes him sick, and then I have to be the one to clean it up." Well, I made the mistake, once, just before sun dance, of eating some fried chicken Lorna had left in the cookshack. By the next day, I was making early and extra trips to the outhouse.

So there was some bad feeling going on related to Lorna. When she stopped by for a visit, though, she'd said the place was looking better than she had ever seen it the whole time Elmer had been living there. Gwen's gardens out back were beginning to provide us with fresh vegetables, mostly greens. After repeated phone calls, we'd finally prevailed on the county, or the tribe, to come out with the big road grader and get the dirt lanes passable to almost any traffic. However, there was still more trouble in paradise. A whispering campaign against Gwen, started by the relatives, had begun. The bad-mouthing mostly took low tacks: One, that she wasn't feeding the old man; she was letting him starve. Two, that she was getting her hands into the old man's finances and embezzling petty cash. It was all projection—accusing her of everything they themselves were guilty of. The result of this was that one of Elmer's daughters was being groomed by various parties to come in and give Gwen and Sage the heave-ho once sun dance was over. The timing was suspect, and we may never know just who was involved or to what extent, but the fact remains that Elmer was always gifted at sun-dance time with food, tools sometimes, and money—and his kids were laying their plans to get their hands on it. That's all there was to it.

But to return to the time just before sun dance, a little before purification was supposed to begin. First to arrive were Dino and some of his relatives. I remember they came in one windy day with Vern Yellowhawk in tow and proceeded to start putting up some of the tipis. I was beginning the last of the mowing—to get the parking and camping areas usable. That evening after supper, and after we'd fed and visited with Grandpa for a while, Gwen said, "Those guys didn't put up the lodges in the right way." Sure enough, two of them blew down in the winds that night. A day or two before purification, I went back to see Elmer about security. I'd already run an idea past him and Gwen—namely, that we use one of Sylvan's drawings—of two crossed *canunpas*—for the poster and T-shirts for this year's sun dance. I had quite a few of Sylvan's drawings by now, all paid for. I'd promised him that I wouldn't use any of them for commercial profit for myself. He'd agreed, and we'd shaken hands. So I'd gone down to the T-shirt printers in Valentine the previous month and also ordered a dozen or so fire-engine-red shirts with "Security" printed on them. I'd gotten a variety of sizes with Sylvan's design and a few words that told the basics: what, when, and where. I ordered almost enough for everybody, as it turned out.

With folks about to come in, we needed to renew the flags, or cloth strips, at the turnoff at the highway and determine the colors for the little strips to be tied around each vehicle antenna after it had been cedared off at the gate. Elmer approved the T-shirt design and told us to use white and green for the antenna flags. I recall going down to the lane just off the road and climbing back up the bank to where the fence met the gateposts to cut off the old, faded red and yellow flags. The day was overcast, but hot and windy. I was on the lookout for snakes—but, all rumors to the contrary, I'd never seen anything worse than a bull snake on the dirt road, much less a rattler. I remember looking around at the vast prairie and feeling good about what I was doing, even if it was so small a thing. Usually it was hard not to feel depressed, what with Elmer's failing health, the stress from the relatives, and all the politicking about who would get Elmer's altar after he kicked the bucket.

Jason had just come in a day or so earlier, and something he'd said had really struck me. We'd been talking about the sun dance, how much longer it would be likely to last, or rather, how many more of them Elmer would be around for. He'd looked me in the eye and said, "This'll be the last." Something told me he was right, but I didn't want to hear it.

Once again, I have to back up and relate some of the events that took place just before the arrivals for purification. Since Norman had taken the originals of Elmer's vehicle titles and other papers, including some potentially relating to ownership of the land he was living on, it seemed he and Gilli were combining to take everything away from the old man. One day, Gwen reminded me that Elmer had told her the spirits had warned him: "Norman's gonna try an' steal the sun dance." On registering the Chev in Elmer's name, there'd been no trouble. But we didn't have the title to the Dodge Ram (that was still in the shop) or the pickup Elmer had given to Gwen. I had gone over to Norman's some weeks earlier and asked for the titles back, but all he would give me were several photocopies of the originals. I was still trying to get the clutch tree on the Ram fixed so they'd have a backup to the Chev, and I didn't want someone else laying claim to it once it was fixed. That issue became moot when it was clear the Ram couldn't be repaired. I had also gone over to Norman's a couple of times trying to get him to do something about Johnson's and Gilli's encroachments on the old man's property and home, but all he did was threaten to come in and "shut that whole sun dance down," which was an empty threat—his way of refusing to do anything. So as sun-dance time grew closer, family tensions were on the rise.

After many calls to the tribal police and, if I recall, a complaint by Gwen to the tribe, we had an official visit one afternoon by some tribal members. They didn't explain exactly who they were to me. Two NDN men came out and asked to speak to Elmer. They talked to Gwen for a while but didn't seem interested in talking to me. I was indoors after lunch, hanging out in the living room, and couldn't help but overhear some of the conversation. Mostly, again, it was in Lakota. I just remember one of the men, who seemed to be in charge, asking something about Gilli.

Elmer's response—"I want Gilli behind me!"—was kind of ambiguous. As far as I know, nothing came of their inquiries. At least, not immediately. However, in a little less than a year's time, there was finally some official action concerning Norman. One thing I'd learned by talking to Gwen and Elmer was that title to the several allotments granted to the Runnings within the reservation were incredibly mixed up, subdivided, and conflicting. Some of the land claimed by the family had been in the name of Elmer's first (and only) wife, Blanche. Some of the lands the (grown) children were living on had been willed to them by her upon her death. As more information emerged, it seemed that Irene had at least a tenuously valid claim on the Ironwood property, although everyone knew she and her outfit were squatting in the home Elmer and Blanche had lived and raised their kids in. And that property, less than a mile from where Elmer's mobile home was now, had been the site of Elmer's first sun dances. Obviously, untangling all this would take years of legal work by

someone familiar with real-estate law as practiced within the reservation system. None of us really had a legal right to keep Gilli
out, although everyone knew he stole, and worse, from the old
man, along with some of the other boys, for drinking money.

Gorgie was coming over more frequently now to visit and to
help out, spelling Gwen. Gwen was upset that the pickup Elmer
had given her was without a title—and hence unregisterable,
thanks to Norman's absconding with the original—and not in
running condition. A fellow she'd called in from Rapid City early
in the spring, one Curtis Milk, had been coming back around
and helping himself to parts from the various vehicles at rest, just
west of the trailer along the fence line. Gwen had called him in to
help her keep the relatives in line. Nearly a full blood, and fluent
in Lakota, he turned out to be a disappointment to her and to all
of us. He'd go back and visit with Elmer, in Lakota, so we never
knew all that was being said. Apparently, he was just talking a
good game, because he was never around to help out with the
work, although he did come around just before sun dance.

Since her pickup was unusable, one day a week or two before
the start of purification, Gorgie came by to sit with Elmer for an
afternoon while I took Gwen vehicle shopping. I felt she deserved
one, after all the work she'd done and all the aggravation she'd
had to go through. We went all the way out to Winner and began
looking over the used vehicles. Nothing came to light at first. We
went farther into town, and I tried to reach the phone number
on a pickup parked on a lawn at a suburban intersection. But
the interior was pretty bad, and Gwen soon decided it wasn't for
her. We also kicked around a secondhand store or two and one
antique shop. Nothing much special was found, and we decided
to try again at another time. Just as we were passing the west
edge of town, however, we passed a used lot / repair shop that
we'd missed on the way in. There, at Winner Auto, we found
what we were looking for. A small pickup, the make I forget, but

with new tires and in good shape. It had been the shop's runner, for whenever they needed to go and pick up a part from NAPA or wherever. The old boy behind the counter said he actually had more into it, what with parts and repairs, than he was asking for it. The price was right, and I paid him then and there. Gwen got the "in transit" tags on, and we drove on home.

By this time, the pups were getting pretty good sized, and Mahto, the black one I was halfway planning on taking home with me, had begun imitating Lala in that he'd begin driving the neighbor's cattle around whenever they'd move down onto our side of the hill. We had to yell at them to get them to stop. The pups were in their "terrible twos" stage of maturity and were deciding when and if they'd listen. But Lala would usually heed me, and they'd follow his lead every time.

One morning, an unfortunate thing happened. As I was leaving my camper, the pups, who spent the nights underneath with Lala and were always happy and playful, jumped up behind me. Just as I stepped off the high rear bumper, Mahto jumped and got clipped a good one under the jaw from my heavily booted foot. He yelped, and I turned and tried to comfort him. I'd felt the unintentional blow and heard him without ever seeing him. It didn't take; from then on, he was wary of me. Only with much coaxing would he come near me anymore. A complete accident, totally unforeseen, but it still makes me sad to think he thought I'd hurt him on purpose.

CHAPTER 24

The Last Go-Round

NOW AND AT LAST, I CAN BEGIN TO RELATE THE EVENTS OF the purification and sun dance. It seemed as if there were a few more people coming in than last year. Even without Nico, Lehr, and my friend Don in Santee, a lot of the old-timers were driving in a few days before purification. Mike Jagod, his wife, Amanda, Sonny, from California; Alan, Steve, and Angie from Michigan; plus, a lot of local folks, including Dino and Sylvan. It seemed that Dino and Gilli had been at pains to entice and enlist sun dancers from among the ranks, and later on, I found out why. In Gilli's case, with his theft of the notebook from 2008, it was pretty obvious. He'd actually called and tried to convince people to come at a later date, which would make them too late for Elmer's sun dance but right on time for his. Irene seemed to be letting him use Elmer's old Ironwood grounds, and even Norman had begun holding one. Gilli had been having one of his own, a few years previously somewhere in the Black Hills, but according to what I'd heard, some warriors from one of the *akicita* societies had come in and shut it down; seems he wasn't doing things right.

But our bunch started pulling together—and since they were, I left. I was so sick of all the drama and the unending rumors and alarms that I actually left a few days before purification began. I had to come back and visit my little dogs and just get some space and quiet. Gwen called often, asking if I was I coming back to dance. I was so burned out, I had to tell her I was undecided at first, and finally, when she tearfully reminded me that this was likely to be the old man's last go-round, I headed back.

Since there'd been many other old-timers around, I wasn't too worried about Gwen not having help while I was gone. Besides, Grandma Darlene Jackson had come from Saint Paul and was so enfeebled by age and illness she mostly had to hang out on the couch. She'd asked me before I left to pick her up some string cheese, and so I stopped at Buche's in Mission, after having stopped in Valentine for the security and memorial T-shirts, and got her some. She was happy to get the cheese, exclaiming, "You remembered!" But Gwen told me later she'd been very needy and demanding.

There was a fellow who came in around the first day of purification who was Gwen's main squeeze, or close enough. At first, I felt a bit jealous, but told myself such feelings were unworthy, especially around sun-dance time. I'd allowed myself to fall into the role of paterfamilias, and those feelings came from that. I can't recall his name, but I didn't want my childishness to cast a pall over the scene or even be noticed. The box of T-shirts was sitting on the kitchen floor, behind the table. This guy was impressed by the design, since, although I'd planned on waiting 'til sun dance was over to give them away as *wopila*, Darlene had begged to be given one right then and there. So just to show myself there were no hard feelings, I offered this friend of Gwen's the original, by Sylvan. He was glad to get it, and I was glad to be able to offer.

A few of Elmer's kids were coming in now that purification was under way. There were a lot of vehicles and tents in the areas I'd been mowing all summer. The two young men from Irene's who'd had the pups follow them over and who'd worked turning Gwen's garden showed back up to do a last-minute mowing

of the westernmost part of the camping area. This may have
occurred just after I returned, on the first day. I recall that when
I got back, the tipis were up, Dino and some other dancers were
arranging for the pine boughs for the arbor to be brought up, and
they were generally getting the dance grounds ready. My prior-
ity was once again setting up the sentry post at the main gate,
getting some cedar, and making some long-handled smudge pots.
Just coffee cans with untwisted coat-hanger wire for handles.
I remember the evening I finished them and was smudging off
vehicles as they came in, wearing my new security T-shirt, those
two young men were using push mowers to finish the camping
area, one long pass after another, and they'd pass each other in
the center of the field. Over and over again, watching them was
almost hypnotic. I was paying them for their time but soon found
there was a rumor going around among the NDN kids that I was
paying people to come and do security. But the crowd of eager
aspirants kinda dwindled when I had to tell them, no, I wasn't
paying for that, just everything else!

Two days later, we set off once again with several pickup
trucks, assorted cars, and a long flatbed trailer to the gravel
road along the stream bottom that flowed just above Crow Dog's.
Above this, and set back a little way, were the old Ironwood
sun-dance grounds, then Irene's, then farther along to Elmer's
dance grounds and the ceremony house / cookshack and Elmer's
mobile home. Across the stream, there were some isolated homes,
then the long stretch of Crow Dog's Paradise. Old Leonard Crow
Dog and one other medicine man—John Around Him, I think
he was called—had consented to lead the dancers, exhort them,
and harangue them during rest breaks. I remember Crow Dog was
walking with us as we'd parked our vehicles, save for the trailer,
some ways back along the road. I was walking a little way behind
him, and Gwen and Sage were a little in front of me. I heard
Gwen tell Sage, "You go and say hello to your grandpa!"

I felt honored just to be walking along the same road as he was, on a beautiful, hot late July afternoon. He'd been the spiritual leader with AIM at Wounded Knee. Some of our leaders had picked out the cottonwood for the sun-dance tree, and after a small girl and boy had swung the axe a stroke apiece, which was almost too heavy for them, the men took turns chopping, until it was almost ready to fall. Then, as before, a line of us took hold and raised our long ash stringers and ranged ourselves beneath the line of fall. We'd notched the back side of the trunk, of course, so that it would fall downhill and out toward the road. The last few blows were struck, and as it fell and we caught it, some of the women began making the brave heart cry.

That, I think was done as if in honoring the fall of an enemy; for there is always danger in a sun dance. Danger since it is such a powerful ceremony, danger in having a hand or arm caught by the tree, danger in offending the spirits, if the tree is allowed to touch the earth at the trunk, and danger to whoever is unwary enough to step over any part of it once it's felled in the right way.

After we'd gotten the tree back to Elmer's, all the vehicles were parked away from the dance circle, except for the flatbed, which was parked off just north of the east gate. All the encircling shade arbor, some six feet across in an enclosure with a diameter of about two hundred feet, had been roofed with the pine boughs. They were also used to enclose three sides of the rest area behind the west gate. The dozens of little painted wooden pegs, which delineated the circle's interior, had been thrust into the ground at the base of the encircling arbor. Every crutch—that is, every forked upright ash support—had gotten a new coat of white paint. The flags of colored cloth were on their staves at each of the four gates, and Elmer's altar was set up just to the left, as one faced to the west gate, which was the entrance to the shade arbor. A large pit in the center of the circle had been dug, with the tools and shovels left strewn about for backfilling. All the pledgers had their ropes and flags and ties ready and waiting in the arbor; putting down one's blanket, or similar, was the way one called one's spot for the next four days. The leaders usually took their places forward in the shade arbor and a little to the left of the entrance as one faced outward.

Now I must back up only a day or two and tell of our last sun-dance meeting. It was a general meeting; all were called to attend. Gwen had gotten Elmer dressed up in his best and wheeled him out onto the front porch to address the group. Earlier in the summer, some group of folks or another, probably local, on hearing poor condition of the *wicasa wakan* following the stroke, had called to announce they were going to do a *heyoka* ceremony (in which, in accordance with tradition, a puppy was to be sacrificed). When Gwen had relayed this to Elmer, he'd reacted strongly: "No! Puppy wants to live!"

A light rain was falling, some of the leaders had spoken already from the encircling arbor; the PA and the mikes and amp for the speakers and drum were set up a little east of the south gate, as usual. So Elmer had to address us in his own voice. All I can remember is that it was the grumpiest I'd ever seen Elmer get. In previous years, he'd call out, "The bear! The bear! The bear is in the camp!" after the second day—meaning his dancers, forbidden the use of water, were starting to smell like an old bear. Or he'd joke about losing his teeth in the dark at 4:00 a.m. and not finding them 'til after the dog had been at 'em, but not now. He just kinda growled at us. I wish there was more, but all I recall is a general taking us to task, which ended with a snarling challenge to any of us to speak and answer him. He posed a specific question or two and challenged us to respond, but no one did. It was obvious he was getting tired of this, but he told us that the spirits had told him that if things were done in the right way, they would give him one more year. It had been common knowledge among those of us who were close to him, and then to all, that he wanted the dancers to stay in the rest arbor all four nights: "No goin' back to camp! We need to do it in the old way!"

Unfortunately, after Gwen had wheeled him back inside, Dino and maybe another leader for the men had gotten on the PA that evening, which followed close on the old man's address, and told us, "Grandpa doesn't want us to suffer; you can go back to your camps at night." Despite that, I was set on trying. But it was getting so cold and damp in there; the weather had briefly relapsed into the springtime pattern. I had a nice fleece blanket with a grizzly on it, and I tried to keep warm in it that first night. But it was too thin; I couldn't stop shivering. I'd gotten it to go up on the hill in, and I'd glad I didn't make the attempt earlier in the year—I'd have frozen.

But back to bringing in the tree. As we got up close to the east gate, having unloaded it from the flatbed and still using the stringers, all the carriers began removing their footwear. No shoes are allowed within a sun-dance circle. I tossed mine off to the south, my left side, as we got close. Once we were in the circle, we rested the butt of the tree in the pit, and then came the round of tying-on—all the ropes above the first crotch, and above them the flags from all the dancers, plus higher the little figure of a man and a buffalo, cut out of rawhide, together with the sun disc. At the base, people were tying on their long strings of prayer ties, so many that it took over half an hour. Then the raising. All the dancers but a few pulled on their ropes from one side and, once the trunk was up, held it there while we fanned out some. Then the dangerous part, the final raising, done slowly so as not to swing it too far to the other side. Once it was upright, we had to move quickly to fan out in an evenly pulling circle. They're never really light, but this was a heavy one. I let my rope go slack just before it reached vertical, for fear of swinging it out too far, and Jason came and pulled on my rope, fearing we wouldn't get it far enough. But the base finally came to rest in the bottom of the pit, and some let go of their ropes and began quickly backfilling. I remember Jason was particularly engaged in digging, throwing the dirt frenziedly with his bare hands while muttering to himself in Lakota. One of the old-time leaders, Dave Sikes, felt he had to speak sharply to get him off the mound so the guys with shovels could get in there.

"Jason!"

"Sorry! I just go into badger mode." *Hoka!*

This was the fourth day of purification, tree day, and the next day would be the first full day of dancing. We'd be up well before sunup to sweat and dance in—but from the moment the tree went up, we were forbidden to eat or touch water. No more optional fasting, and (supposedly) no going back to our individual camps at night. Before that, we still had one more night in camp, but first I had to recover my shoes. I walked around the outside of the arbor on the north side and began looking for them. They weren't where I looked to find them, so I went a little farther south. The farther across the east gateway I went, the more I began to feel I should retrace my steps and go all the way around, come up from the south side, and get them from there; but I was so tired. Someone even hollered at me, "Karl! Don't cross the east gate!"

"I'm not!" I yelled back, but I was, in fact, nearly all the way across before I found my shoes. And, during the dance, I was to pay for it.

It was strange; during my first dances at Santee, I'd been so overawed at the prospect of actually being allowed to participate that I had a positive fear of making mistakes—and crossing the east gate after the tree was up was foremost among them. So it was with a sense of foreboding disquiet that I returned to my camper van that evening.

One last issue with Gwen and the relatives. Just before sun dance, she and I had posted a set of rules by the front door. These were designed to keep the family from taking too much advantage of the old man and his things. The usual rules about no alcohol, drugs, cameras, guns, or animals were already up at the main gate on the dirt lane. I understood her frustration with having folks come traipsing in and making free with the household. For instance, during the last woodcutting and mowing during purification, everyone who needed gas for their chainsaw or mower would come into the shop shed and help themselves. I'd have had no problem with that, except the little spouts, held in place by the cans' caps, were fitted to each one. But no one paid any attention to keeping the right spout on the right can, so by the fourth day you couldn't pour out any fuel without the mismatched cans and spouts leaking all over the place. Since there were five or six different ones, finding the right spout was impossible without investing an hour or so just doing that. It's frustrating to have the care one has taken, even in so small a thing, spoiled by carelessness, and Gwen felt the same way about the interior of the mobile home. People would come in, eat, smoke, wash their hands in the kitchen sink, have coffee, and leave their mugs out in the living room—and guess who'd have to clean up, on top of being a twenty-four-hour caregiver? Gwen's control issues may have been a little sharper than most, but then she was doing more than most, and even Patti had gotten on my case about leaving coffee cups out in the yard at Santee.

One of the new posted rules was that no one was to bring in their laundry to do in Elmer's machines. Gwen had told me certain relatives had been known to come in and overload the washer and dryer. Perhaps that's why the old dryer had been shrieking so badly. Plus, they'd use up all the detergent and head off without so much as a thank-you. So during purification, when some relatives had left a big bag of their dirty laundry at the front door, Gwen told me who'd done it, where their tent was, and asked me to return it to them. This I did, feeling a little caught in the middle again, but luckily they weren't at home. So I just left it at their door, or in this case, flap.

Elmer had so many grown kids that I couldn't keep track of them all. Gwen, having spent the winter with Webster, Gilli, and Anthony (or Iktomi) and his woman, knew them all pretty well, at least by name. There were a number of daughters, Martina in particular, as well. I did know her. She'd shown up one day with a boyfriend, or her husband. I'd met her before, and I knew she made and sold star quilts. She kind of put me off because the last time she'd come around, she'd jumped out of her vehicle as soon as it stopped in the drive, got out her catalogue of quilts, and asked me without a handshake or even a hello if there was one I wanted to buy! As it turned out, there was; but she made her sale, came in and said hello to her father, and just hit the road again. Of all Elmer's relatives, his brother, Al, was the only one I had any respect for.

Things were starting to move pretty fast just before and during purification. There were a number of young men and women coming in to help out, and I handed out nearly all the security T-shirts. We had the smudge cans going at the gate and the strips of cloth to tie around each aerial. I'd even gotten a couple of handheld CB walkie-talkies, but there was little need for them. The drive in from the highway to Elmer's was so long and the final approach down the hill so open that anyone coming in was obvious. There were no other approaches to the property, except for the little trail that led up the hill to the east toward Irene's and the old Ironwood grounds. All in all, the change was pretty dramatic. From months of little to no company, apart from Sylvan and his clan and unwelcome visits by the relatives—which I don't really count as companionable—to a mini village of a couple of hundred souls, all in the space of a week or so. The young people who were volunteering for security at the gate were pretty gung-ho. There was a healthy contingent of women over at the cookshack, and all were coming in to see Elmer for a hand-shake and a visit, so a lot of the stress was off Gwen to always have to be there for him.

I recall the evening the tree went up, one of the young men on the gate (who seemed slightly in awe of me, which I found unfathomable) mentioned that he had no T-shirt for his gate duty. So I gave him the last of the spare security T-shirts. By now, the sweat-lodge fires had been going morning and evening for days. A dozen or more tipis were up, not counting Elmer's two, one for the dancers' *canunpas* to sleep in, one for hospitality. And the entire forty-acre field north and west of the sun-dance grounds were covered with pop-up tents, and vehicles of every description parked behind them along the western fence line. The drummers and singers were getting in voice, and everything seemed to be going well. No owls this year!

One of the sun dancers, Mike from Michigan, who with his wife, Amanda, had given Grandma Darlene a ride back to the Twin Cities the year before, was a cheerful, willing soul. We'd hit it off the year before, and now, with Mahto getting so big and aggro, I was having doubts about how he'd fit in with my crew of shih tzus. Mike said he'd been wishing he could get a real rez dog to take home, and although Sage acted a bit peeved about it the next day, I got out Mahto's immunization record and the heartworm medicine I'd bought for him and told Mike he was OK to go home with them. Turns out he wasn't a bit of trouble on the way back and has turned out to be a really good dog for them. It was a wrench and no mistake when they left, but it worked out well. Mike liked the name, which was good, since Mahto had begun to answer to it, and one can't simply change a dog's name; it confuses 'em.

Jason was in his element as fire keeper, tending the rocks being cooked for sweat. He had these enormous leather gauntlets he'd wear whilst pitch-forking the hot grandfathers into the lodge, and the next morning, after we'd all gone back to our camps anyhow, at about 4:30 a.m., his shrill tenor yawp split the prairie night once again: "*Hoka hey,* sun dancers! The grandfathers are waiting!" I'd once overheard him relate how, years ago, he'd told Elmer he wanted to be the camp crier.

I was already awake when I heard him. I'd gotten up at about four and had some warmed-over coffee I'd taken the precaution of making the night before. Coffee had always been allowed at Elmer's sun dance, as long as it was taken before being sweated in. After that, nothing all day. The only thing that worried me was the condensation on the creamer bottle. Since I wasn't supposed to touch water for four days, it bothered me that the drops had gotten on my hand again!

Like the other dancers, I had all my gear ready—the flags, rope, and ties were already on the tree, and I had my sage cuffs and anklets and crown, wrapped with red cloth, and I had my fan and skirt. There was beginning to be the faintest suggestion of light in the east as I barefooted it across the yard to the lodge fire. My bear fleece was laid out in the arbor, so I had my place set. The night air was cold as we waited our turn to sweat in. I also had my towel, wrapped around my shoulders, for the sweat and drying off afterward. I'd chosen a big one and hugged it around my chest and shoulders for warmth. Even so, sitting on a bench close to the fire, your backside would freeze while your front would roast. There was a little talk and laughter among the dancers, but mostly I looked up at the stars that first morning. We were so far away from any large cities or towns that the Milky Way was clearly visible. Perhaps I was wrong when I said earlier that I was dancing for Leonard Peltier's parole from prison in 2008. It seems to me now that it was 2009 when he came up for it one last time, and it was denied again, although everyone knows he's innocent.

Finally, our turns came, and we all went into the little lodge. I say *all*, but some were in ahead, and a few groups were still waiting. As I bent down low, I could hear the women's voices raised in song from the women's lodge, well away on the other side of the sweat-lodge circle. We kept silence as the grandfathers passed in, then sang our songs and prayed. Since this was a different sweat to one preceding a doctoring ceremony, only seven stones were used, and there were no second, third, or fourth rounds, and no prayers were made with the pipe.

Speaking of which, we all had our *canunpas* waiting for us in the tipi, and after we were dried off, we went in to get them. You had to remember where yours had been placed against the low racks the night before, after the tree had gone up, since there was almost no light by which to see.

This done, we began lining up on the north side of the arbor with the leaders opposite the north gate; at least I believe so. Not wearing my contacts or hearing aids, some details always escape me. It's hard to describe the anticipation, the real sensation of awe as one awaits the first blast from the eagle-bone whistle. I remember the morning star shining brightly above us. Then it came, the signal, and we turned to pray to the west. Again, and we advanced a short way, and prayed to the north. Again, and we advanced a ways farther, stopped, and turned to the east. Once more, and we went a little ways and stopped for the south. Then the last whistle came, and we filed in through the east gate, being cedared off as we passed through, between the flags, and turning again in a full circle as we began dancing in.

We danced to the positions we were to take for the duration of the ceremony, with the leaders directing us to an even spacing. The drumming and the singers had begun as we entered and were getting into voice with the first of the songs. Apart from the taboo on telling too much of what specifically goes on within that circle, I may say that the first round consists of the dancers, on another signal, rushing in groups to press the stems of their pipes against the base of the tree, fanning the tree with their eagle-wing fans, and making their personal supplications. One is supposed to take nothing in, besides one's *canunpa*, to get one through the four days.

After this, the dancers resume their places, once again honor the four directions, then the leaders direct all the dancers to proceed to place their *canunpas* on another low rack to the south of the altar, which is itself set up just to the south of the west gate, the entrance to the rest arbor. Well, we danced around that circle four times, made a rush at the tree with our pipes, made our prayers, and set our pipes up. The sun was well up by now, as we'd made our entrance just as it rose above the horizon, but the sky was gray and the air very cool. We'd resumed our places, danced a bit more, then filed into the rest arbor. The lone, brave young man who'd stayed there all night was looking kinda beat. I huddled into my fleece in a nearly silent blur of a world. Only those within a few feet of me were distinguishable, either by sight or voice. We waited, rested, and waited some more. Too long! Something was wrong. I had no idea what was happening until finally Elmer came out in his wheelchair and got after us. On the PA, I could hear him well enough. Apparently, an hour or more had passed since our first round. "Why ain't you guys dancin'?" he demanded. "You should be on the second or third round by now!"

He was really mad, and I didn't learn why until later. Apparently, one of the two senior men's leaders, David, had left and gone into town after we'd gone in to rest, quite against the rules, and Dino and the others hadn't been willing to start again until he got back. No reason for it that I ever heard—just a very bad start and things not being done the right way.

The rest of the first day stayed cool, though the sun finally came out later in the afternoon, just before we sweated out, racked our pipes, and went back to camp. As I've said, no one was staying in the arbor all night, except for that one standout young man. I worried about this then and still feel bad about it. He was the one who, earlier in the summer, had come in to *opagi* Elmer for sun dance while I was out; Gwen later told me he'd done so very beautifully. He was also the one she named to the old man when he asked her if she thought there was anyone walking in a good enough way to take "that suitcase," after he "kicked the bucket."

The old yellow suitcase, which was usually kept locked in the school bus, contained his altar, rattles for doctoring, and medicines. She told me that when he'd asked, she'd thought it over, and the only person who came to mind was this young man. He looked to be a *wasicu*, but he may have had some Native heritage for all I know. He reminded me a bit of how I'd been at first, at Santee before Patti's lies and abuse, and before my own drinking and the sunstroke in 2001 had taken the edge off my dedication and humility.

I'd also had a little more than I could take of some NDNs' attitudes. Once early in 2001, I'd been visiting Elmer for a while, and another Indian man had been there. Elmer had misplaced something—I can't recall what. I jumped up from my chair in the living room to help look for it. For some reason this struck the other visitor as wormy or somehow otherwise unpalatable. He'd been polite enough, at first, shaken hands, but after I began to help in the search, I noticed from the tail of my eye a look of undisguised contempt directed at me. Was I too eager? Who could know? Just him, and he wasn't sayin'. At the time, I wanted to light into him, especially since he wasn't helping to look, but I kept it zipped. Wasn't gonna start no ruction in a holy man's house. I figured whatever it was, it was his problem, not mine, but it still rankled. I'd also begun to feel that, no matter how hard I worked or how much I helped out with the food, gas, bills, and errands, it would never be enough. I would always be just another *wasicu*. This, too, had dulled the edge of my enthusiasm.

Gwen had told me that she knew Elmer was concerned over who would get that suitcase, and he thought about it a lot. Contrary to my previous understanding, whoever had it, it seems, would be able to call the spirits. As he'd told us at ceremony at the new house in Santee, "The spirits, sometimes when they come in, they tell me, 'We're going to mess with that person!' I always tell 'em, 'No, don't do it.'" Apparently, in the wrong hands, the power of such an altar can be abused. This, I think, was what worried the old man so much.

Nonetheless, when the spirits had come in and pounded on the floor of my little upstairs prayer room, back in 2008, I'd answered the call even though I'd been a little spooked by it. I put down the bottle for good, picked up the pipe again, and come back—and I'm so grateful that despite my many shortcomings, they'd found me worthy to serve. Now, however, even after all my work, I'd made the mistake of going too far across the east gate after the tree was up.

The second day's dancing had gone better. Everybody stayed in camp, there were no incidents I was aware of, and by mid-morning, we were starting to dance hard. The chorus of eagle-bone whistles was alternating back and forth, from one side of the circle to the other, providing a sort of high end of prayer as the drummers and singers kept the beat. Ordinarily, as I've said, I wouldn't report anything that took place within that circle except my own experiences, but if this is to be a more or less complete memoir, I need to add a little.

I'd decided not to pierce on the third day, the healing round, but during the first piercing round on the second day. This was about midmorning. Dino was in charge of the piercings again, so I told him that I was intending to do it then. When I was able to make out, from my place just past the south gate, that the pledger ahead of me had broken and danced back, I turned around and ran around the circle once, to take my place. I lay down on the buffalo robe and pointed to where my pins were stuck in my sage crown, when asked. One always forgets, until the moment, how much it hurts when the pins go in. I made my way to the tree, prayed, and danced until I broke free. The helper took hold of my right sage cuff and danced us around the circle, with an honoring spin at each of the gates. The first was at the west gate, just behind where the robe lay. As I whirled in place, I felt something go *pop!* under my left kneecap! Each step from then on taken with that leg and incorporating any kind of turn was just excruciating. It's a wonder I stayed upright. I could dance in place and when moving in a more or less straight line, but I'd apparently blown out one of the big side tendons that stabilizes the joint when turning. I was lucky; that's probably one of the least of the things that could happen when one disrespects the spirits, however unintentionally, by going too far across the east gate. Lucky, I mean, that I was able to finish the dance. The next two and a half days were kinda rough, but it was just one more pain to endure, to dedicate to Wakan Tanka. I was grateful for it!

That wasn't the only memorable thing that happened. The healing round took place on the afternoon of the third day, as it usually had. After nearly a full day's dancing, it was always the last round—and afterward, all those who had come to support, or those who'd attended and wished a blessing, would line up on the south side of the arbor, outside, holding a sprig of sage. They were allowed inside the arbor, to embrace the tree and make their prayers. Afterward, when the line had reformed and the sun dancers were exiting the east gate, we proceeded past all those present and shook hands. I had heard many people say that the spirits of Elmer's altar were powerful, and I'd seen something of this myself in previous sun dances. In each of them, during the healing round, a fog had come up. A cool, white mist would form out of nowhere, no matter how fiery the day had been, and envelop the entire circle, so that nothing beyond a few yards was even visible. Four times I'd seen this happen—in Nebraska and South Dakota in August, when I would have sworn there wasn't a drop of moisture in the air. I knew better than to start asking questions about such a thing, so I was left with what Elmer'd call "my own mind" for an answer. I think the spirits brought that mist in when they came in to do their doctoring; perhaps it was how they did it. Perhaps it was a cloak for their presence. But this year, there was no mist during the healing round.

As I say, I'd heard extraordinary accounts of the spirits' power at Elmer's sun dance. Lightning striking nearby out of a clear blue sky at Santee. The woman who was unable to conceive a child until she came to sun dance and prayed, and then she had a baby the following year. Not to mention the little Kiowa baby girl my ex and I had danced for in my first year. Her excess cerebral-spinal fluid had simply gone away, and her spina bifida had completely healed up by the time we got back from Santee to Alabama.

But I'd also heard of signs of the power waning. Dave Ross, who'd been my friend back in Santee, had been so disheartened back at the dance in 1999 when he saw the leaves on the sun-dance tree beginning to wither and fade. He'd said, "The leaves on Elmer's tree never used to do that; they used to stay fresh and green all four days." Gorgie and Gwen and I had tried to contact Dave and as many of the other old-timers as we could, both to prevent Gilli's attempted forestalling of his dad's dance and to call in everyone who might want to come. We looked for him on Facebook and couldn't find him. Now it seemed the power was failing even more.

During purification, especially just before the tree went up, different people would get on the PA. There was a separate microphone, so people could address the dancers and support-ers. Various people spoke, including Dino, the older *wicasa wakan* who harangued us, and a Lakota woman named Marie

Whirlwind Soldier. She'd been very hard on Gwen the previous year, and now it seemed the Dino-led cabal had recruited her. She got up and spoke about all the hard work Sylvan had done to create such a beautiful arbor and sun-dance grounds. No mention of Yellowhawk or me. She also spoke about how wrong it was to allow white people at the sun dance, "stealing our ceremonies, so there won't be anything left for our grandchildren." I was taken aback at this, but I didn't say anything. I'd been present at the medicine men's gathering back in 2000 or 2001, when Elmer had addressed the group: "When the spirits told me to put up a sun-dance grounds for the people, they didn't say just for the Indian people." And not a single *wicasa wakan* there had taken issue with him. He'd specifically pointed me out as a non-Indian sun dancer of his, adding, "I keep one o' them with me all the time."

As it turned out, there was a faction led by Dino and Norman, which seemed to include Marie, Lorna, Sylvan, and Vern Yellowhawk. They simply didn't care that the old man had given the latter part of his life to trying to keep alive the ways and ceremonies of his people, and they surely no longer regarded anything he had to say. It was about this time, too, that we began hearing rumors that Elmer's daughter Martina was being groomed to come in and replace Gwen as Elmer's caretaker, no matter that the old man had appointed Gwen at the spirits' direction.

It seemed that all the work and care that Gwen, Gorgie, Jason, Konda, and a few others had done to keep things good for the old man was being swept away and ignored—mostly by, and for the benefit of, the Dino-led faction. It's hard to know what exactly was happening, since they obviously weren't telling us about their plans, but Gwen heard a rumor going around that she wasn't feeding Elmer and was stealing from him. Martina began calling and declaring that she'd be coming to take over the old man's caretaking after sun dance. I suspect that the visit from the men from the tribal advocates was a result of this. They'd asked Elmer about who he wanted with him, and he'd said, "I want my family with me." This was told to Gwen by Curtis Milk, who spoke Lakota. Martina and her backers took this to mean that he wanted her. But, as Jason reminded Gwen, "How many times has Grandpa told you that you're part of his family?"

Grandpa had told everyone who he wanted for his cook and housekeeper way back before his stroke. Then, after the relatives had driven Gwen out the previous winter, they'd completely failed to care for him. He'd also had a dream, just before the stroke, about using only seven stones in the ceremony sweat, but Dino had gone ahead and used the traditional twenty-four. Gwen flat-out blamed Dino for the stroke as a result of ignoring Elmer's dream. Later on, a month or so after the sun dance, an old-timer called Leonard Young had called and asked Gwen what Dino had had to do with Elmer's stroke.

Gwen asked, "How do you know he had anything to do with it?"

"Every time something's happened to Elmer," Leonard replied, "Dino's always had something to do with it."

So that was the lay of the land as the fourth day began. As we were sitting in the shade arbor during one of the breaks, one of the guys asked me what had become of that fellow who was with me last year, that White Hawk. I explained about having had to change my plans about having him stay over the winter at my little place in Minnesota. About how he'd found a girlfriend and, having been so hot to get a few push-ups in one time before she arrived to pick him up, that he'd pushed a plugged-in electric space heater right up against a stack of record albums without paying the slightest attention to whether or not it was turned on. How he'd also neglected to put it back when her car showed up but had hurried his shirt on and out the door. At that point, I explained, I realized he was a fire hazard. I noticed a few of the men were paying close attention to what I was saying, but it seemed to satisfy, especially when I added, "When he came to pick up his stuff, he was driving her car, so at least he had somewhere to go."

That last day, given what had been said by Marie Whirlwind Soldier and the reappearance of Sylvan and Vern in Dino's camp and the pain in my knee, I was having a hard time concentrating on my prayers with a good heart. I remember feeling so low at one point, I completely offered myself to Tunkasila: "Oh, just take me now, Grandfather." That didn't happen, obviously, but the *heyokas* did get after me worse than ever. Two of those contraries, the sacred clowns in their ragged, short, black jeans and hoods and paint came around the circle, as they do every year, to tease and test the dancers' dedication. Pulling faces, holding up a dipper and bucket of water right in my face, letting it pour out in front of me, which was par for the course. And then going a step beyond the usual and dancing around behind me and getting hold of the top of my skirt and miming the act of pouring the water down my rear end. Admittedly, I couldn't ever see much in the circle without my contacts. Everything past ten feet to either side was just a blur of shapes and colors, but I'd still never seen them do that to anyone! Maybe it was my long blond hair, I don't know. I do know a couple of Lakota ladies behind me thought it was pretty funny; I could hear them laughing over the singers and the drum.

But still that wasn't the worst. I can't recall much of the dance's end. With my knee, I wasn't much help in taking the tree down or in removing the pine boughs from the arbor. After sweating out for the first time and changing, the usual feast and giveaways were pretty fine. I recall sitting down next to a young Lakota lady and comparing notes on how it was to fast all four days. At some point, I went into the trailer and sat down gingerly in an armchair and explained to those present what had happened to my knee. A young white woman exclaimed, "I know! I was there when it happened!" She tried to do some of that Reiki energy healing on it; don't know if that helped any.

People seemed more intent than usual on taking some of the leaves and branches from the tree. A week later, I was still cleaning up the grounds and burning odds and ends and branches left behind in the sweat-lodge fire. The worst was, after the feast and giveaways, almost everyone left immediately. There was a long line of vehicles heading up the hill and out. Gwen later told me she'd been in back with Elmer, and he'd said, "They're all goin' home." But not everyone hightailed it. A few folks—Lorna, Gorgie, and one or two of the other dancers—stayed to help clean up. The campground was a shambles, however, and I had to pack a lot of the left-behinds out to the big Dumpster by the front gate. There were some good ground scores, however. I remember coming onto a whole handful of sweet-grass braids. I picked up a very nice woolen purple blanket, but felt I should ask someone about it. Lorna was over at the cookshack, helping clean up and organize the leftover foodstuffs securely so Elmer would have them and they wouldn't walk away. A couple of his boys, Webster and another, were taking the boughs off the arbor. I walked over to the picnic tables as Lorna was coming out of the kitchen.

"Lorna," I said, "I found this nice blanket over in the camping area. You don't know who it might belong to, do you?"

"No, Karl, but if you want it, you should go ahead and keep it. You've done so much out here!"

That was good to hear. I made the mistake of mentioning Gwen's name in connection with whatever it was we'd discussed next; I saw her eyes narrow, her lips compress, and her head go back just a little. All the signs of anger. It seemed as if only Gorgie, myself, Jason and Konda, and a few others wanted to respect Gwen for all she'd done for the old man.

But to return briefly to the last events of the fourth day, directly after we'd charged out of the east gate for the last time and cleaned up a bit, and I changed, there was the feasting. Hot dogs, hamburgers on fry bread, salads, watermelon, and lots of soda and coffee. Then people reassembled around and inside the circle for the *wopila*, or thanksgiving, giveaway. I had a few things to give. But I'd given Gwen the commemorative T-shirts so she could be the one giving them away to the people and so be due an honoring. Just before they were all gone, Sylvan came over and asked if he could get one. He'd been sitting over on the north side with Dino and the rest of 'em, and I noticed him looking a little uncertain and apprehensive, as if he realized he'd gotten pretty involved with a bunch of new people he suddenly wasn't too sure of. Of course we gave him one—it was his artwork on the front! The German contingent, Ulee and his wife, and the others (whose names always escape me) also had some commemorative T-shirts and caps, plus some copies of snapshots of Grandpa, the grounds with tipis up, and a beautiful evening shot of the tipi poles silhouetted against the sky. Really beautiful. They'd been coming across the pond since before my time at Santee.

When we finally did the giveaway, I went over to the drum, which was then being manned by Gilli and Webster and one or two others, and put some money and tobacco on the drum and asked them for an honoring song for Gwen. I got on the PA for the first and only time and announced the honoring, mentioning how she had worked so hard and done such a good job of taking care of Grandpa since his stroke. We were sitting on the south side of the arbor, east of the drum, which was nearby the south gate, where it always was. I returned to our place, feeling extremely self-conscious, and as the song began, I draped a brain-tanned elk hide across her shoulders and then gave her a special necklace I'd made. Native-style bead necklaces had been a thing of mine ever since my days working on the powwow trail in the Southeast. This time I'd put together a humdinger, if I say so myself. The centerpiece was a polished spiny oyster half shell, a brilliant red. Then came alternating antique purple chevron beads, large ones, and round coral root. Nice Kingman turquoises and smaller corals and turquoises.

After I'd nervously fumbled it on, we shook hands, and I sat down, relieved to be out of the spotlight. People began coming up to get a shirt, and I chanced to look over at the drummers: Web and Gilli both had real sour looks, like they'd just bitten a lemon. I remarked to Gwen later on that I wasn't altogether upset by the fact that, under the circumstances, they were obliged to honor her after they'd both given her such a hard time. Sylvan had gotten his shirt and was sitting over with Dino and Marie, still not looking too happy about getting caught up in the politics without even realizing it.

A few of the sun dancers and supporters had brought gifts for Gwen and Sage. Just before sun dance, I'd taken Sage into Mission, at Gwen's request, and gotten him some new clothes and shoes. It was a shame that she had to ask, although I was glad to help. She should have gotten her promised raises, and she should have had a regular relief to give her some time off, but I never saw or heard of these things happening. I'd been getting burned out myself, even before sun dance, and I was only the helper's helper! I remember now that it seemed as if there were whole stretches of time when not much was going on, but then I recall that it was rare to have a single day go by without some kind of stupid drama, usually involving one or another of his kids. One of the things Grandpa told Sage was, "After I kick the bucket, I'm always gonna be around with you." Or something very like that, anyway. It seemed to echo what he'd reported one of his helping spirits had said to him all those years ago, when they'd first given him his altar: "Hey, I'm gon' be you buddy. I'll stick around you all the time."

Gwen told me he'd also said to all the participants at the last monthly ceremony, "Stock up on food and water. Them places, like New York an' Washington, they're gonna be just flat! And underwater." Later on, he'd elaborated on this to Gwen, after he'd recovered from his stroke, thanks to her nursing and ministrations: "There's gonna be a hurricane," he'd said, "big enough to reach up here!"

"Do you mean a tornado, Grandpa?"

"No, goddamn it, I mean a hurricane!"

I was able to stay on a week for so after sun dance. To back up a little, the first day after the tree was down, I couldn't do much, on account of my knee. I remember being in the living room with Gwen and a few others and explaining how and when, if not why, I'd blown it out. Turns out Gwen had come into the circle to support me when I pierced and had been right behind me. Maybe Sage was too; I don't recall. In a day or two, I was able to get around fairly well.

A few days later, Jason and Konda, the relatives, and the last of the sun dancers and supporters who'd stayed on left, and it was once again down to Gwen, Elmer, Sage, and myself. Mike Jagod had taken Mahto with him, so we only had Dakota, Hokshila, the little cat, and the chickens. Dino and his outfit had at least taken down the tipis and stored them with their ropes and stakes and flap pins in the garbage cans in which they were kept. Jason had done a lot to help pack up the rest of the sundance gear and lock it all with Elmer's suitcase in the school bus. For a day or two, maybe, we had quiet. There was no need for me to keep the grounds trim; the scores of feet and the multitudes of vehicles had flattened the camping and parking areas, as well as around the cookshack. And for once, the tribal garbage pickup was more or less timely. There were lots of extra bags sitting around the Dumpster, but they came and picked them up. I believe I made at least one last trip into Mission, picked up on some more CDs at White Horse (which one simply couldn't find elsewhere), groceries and gas, and another basket of chicken strips for Elmer.

I think it was after this trip that I made the mistake of leaving him alone to eat, and he just inhaled it, choked, and got me back in there on the run! I remember it took him a while to clear his airway, coughing, and I was in a sweat until he got the last of it down and started breathing normally again. I was in mortal dread of what Gwen might have had to say to me if she'd come back in just then. But it passed, and I sat with him. I held his mug of green tea (with a straw, so he could drink it more easily) and helped him finish his lunch more slowly. He was getting a little more strength in his right hand and arm, but the left side was still totally without motor control.

Gwen was getting more and more calls from Martina. She was becoming insistent about coming in and "taking care of my dad." The utterly false accusations about Gwen were still flying around among the rest of the family, as far as we could make out. Curtis, who had come earlier in the spring in response to Gwen's call for help, was back and around the place on and off. He said he was working on the pickups for Elmer, the ones along the fence line that didn't run, but all he did was take parts off the one Elmer had given to Gwen the year before and use them himself. With his knowledge of Lakota, he said that Elmer had told the men from Elderly Assistance that he "wanted his family around him" and that the family were using that to kick Gwen and Sage to the curb.

Gwen had already warned Martina off, telling her, "If you come in here and take over, it won't be long before Gilli'll be back and stealing Elmer's things for booze money."

"Oh no!" Martina had replied. "I won't let Gilli do that."

Finally, the day came when I had to leave. My little dogs and cat had been boarded for two and a half months, and it wasn't fair to them to leave 'em any longer. Since then, I've wondered many times if I did the right thing. There had been talk of one of the local sun dancers, or Jason, or someone coming in to offer Gwen some backup against the relatives. Gwen kept me posted by phone. About a week after I left, Gwen called me up one afternoon to tell me she'd just had to give the bad news that they'd missed sun dance to several carloads of would-be sun dancers and supporters. They'd arrived that afternoon looking to set up camp, *opagi* Elmer, and sun dance. They were the folks on the stolen list that Gilli had reached but we hadn't. Gwen said she'd explained to them about the stolen address book, but it was pretty cold comfort. One fellow in particular had been upset: "I've spent a thousand dollars to come here!" Nonetheless, she told them they had to turn around and head home.

The next thing was about two weeks after that. It seemed Martina was finally making good on her threats to come in and take over Elmer's care. Gwen had said repeatedly, "Once she gets here and finds out how much work it is to take care of Grandpa, she won't want to do it."

It fell out that Martina showed up one afternoon, marched in there, and just began shoving Gwen out of the way. She (apparently) told her kids to tear up the flower beds Gwen had planted around the front porch, for which I'd built the retainers. Her kids were just as heedless and unmannered as possible. They were all over the new furniture I'd bought for everyone, spilling soda and snacks, and generally trashing the place. Gwen hung in as long as she could, but finally one day, she came back out into the living room after seeing to Grandpa, and there was Webster, sitting in the easy chair and fooling around with a big knife in a meaningful way. She quickly found someone to tow her little trailer to a lot in Mission and moved herself, Sage, and Dakota there. This must have been around the end of August.

CHAPTER 25

The Final Call

ONE THING I HAVE RECALLED OFTEN WAS THE LAST SWEAT AT Elmer's place. I had smoked the pipe I'd loaded for sun dance within the four days afterward, but one more sweat for giving thanks was in order. As it turned out, the only other ones to come in with me then were Gilli and Webster. This was within a week after sun dance, so Gwen was still there, and I believe Jason kept fire and ran the door. He did a lot of fire-pit maintenance. Well, we got in there, and Gilli was running it. We went through the songs and the four doors, but I hadn't memorized all the songs too well. Those two never said anything to me, but from their looks and their whole demeanor, the message was obvious: "We're the Indians here, not you. This is ours, not yours." It was in the air pretty heavy. Even some of the sweats in Santee, and at Rosebud in 2000, when I couldn't make it all the way through, weren't as bad as this one. I knew they were robbing their own father and debasing their own people's ceremonies by carrying the pipe while drinking and drugging—and I knew they knew I knew, and they didn't care. My very first impression of Gilli had been of a vulture circling, just waiting to land and feed, as I'd told to Dave Ross so long ago in Santee. Now the buzzards had landed.

Two weeks after Martina and Web finally succeeded in driving Gwen out, she called me. She was crying. "Karl," she sobbed, "Elmer's dead. They said he had a heart attack. They took him to the hospital, and he was DOA." I sat there too stunned to speak at first. I can't recall a thing I said. I know I asked her what happened. Then as my wits slowly returned, I muttered something like, "Well, it didn't take them long to get what they wanted, did it? You kept him going for a year, but he only lasted a couple weeks with them." She told me when the funeral was going to be, and I made arrangements with my neighbors to come over and care for my animals while I was gone.

When I got back, there were a lot of vehicles parked over by the cookshack and ceremony house. As I came up to the main gate at the bottom of the long hill, I noticed a couple of things. One was that the new washer was sitting out by the Dumpster. The other was that one or more Indian kids had a fire going in the backyard, right where the Chev used to be. It wasn't in sight now. I saw one of the kids make a couple of trips into the back door, emerging each time with a bundle of papers. Elmer's papers. He kept a second suitcase of property documents, copies of treaties, and other important stuff—including photos of old-time Indians from whom he and his family were descended. Now, doubtless under one of the adults' direction, it was all going into the flames. Doubtless, again, so that no adult could be charged or implicated in any ensuing legal implications. The sight of it made me sick.

When I got into the mobile home, it was like stepping into a strange house. The dogs were gone (not that they'd ever been allowed inside), the new furniture was gone, the beautiful hand-painted buffalo skull Elmer had kept hanging on the west wall of the living room was gone, and there stood Elmer's boys, Webster and Norman, and Shannon and Web's wife, lining up to shake hands with shit-eating grins on their faces. I left quickly and went over to the ceremony house. There were a lot of folks there

already. As I got close, Gilli came out and shook hands with
me, then hurried away. I turned away, wiping off my hand on
the thigh of my jeans, and went inside. There were the kitchen
chairs. Tables were being set up buffet-style, and the big coffee
urn from the cookshack was being run by several women. I saw
that the door between the two rooms was open, and there, on a
buffalo robe, inside a beautiful star quilt, on a covered trestle, lay
Elmer's body. I went over, took a look, and started crying. I left
the ceremony house and quickly walked around the corner to the
empty south side until I was done.

I went back in later. Dino had been in touch with me about
a fellow who'd beaded the soles of the ceremonial moccasins for
Elmer and needed to be paid. He handed the mocs to Dino as
soon as I handed him the money. Looked like a good job to me.
There were programs for the service, and I saw I'd been listed
as an honorary pallbearer. Two medicine men— Leonard Crow
Dog and a Mr. Around Him—would run the service, deliver
the eulogy, generally address us, and see to the distribution of
Elmer's ceremonial possessions among his sons. There was to be
a dance of the sun dancers in the circle the next morning before
the burial, and I needed to get an eagle-bone whistle. I talked to
Gwen about it after she and Sage came up to the trailer. After cir-
culating a bit, we left and went back to the little in-town trailer
park in Mission, where they were living. On our way, she tried
calling Nico to see if he had a whistle I might borrow, but when
she reached him, all he'd say was, "I'm not at home."

There was, luckily, a spare site at the trailer park where I
could park my camper van and get power in. I visited with the
couple who owned and ran the place, and they seemed decent
enough. Gwen's trailer was pretty small, but it seemed she and
Sage were managing. I know Sage was glad to get away from
Grandpa's, since he now had some friends his own age to play

with. I can't recall too many details of that evening, but it seems we had dinner together and called it a night.

The next morning was warm and bright. Gwen and I got to Elmer's about nine-ish. Months earlier, he'd told Gwen, "When I kick the bucket, you gonna have to put on a dress and feed all my sun dancers." She had brought a lot of food, cake, and other things. I was also remembering what he'd said about getting the sun-dance grounds looking nice, because there were to be a lot of people at his funeral. Looking out over the grounds, where the vehicles were again filling the parking areas, at least one tipi was back up, and a number of folks had camped out overnight. I was glad Sylvan and Marie had managed to get the outhouses and the uprights in the arbor painted so that it did present well.

The cookshack was open for business by the time we got there, and there was fry bread and coffee for all. Inside the ceremony house, Elmer's casket was still against the east wall, but closed now. There had been a large glass bowl filled with filter cigarettes free for anyone, but it was gone. All the previous afternoon, except when we'd shaken hands, I never saw Gilli. Everyone else was around, even Jamie Chinana from Santee and the famous *heyoka* who was in *Wayne's World II*, but I never laid eyes on Gilli that day, except when the eagle headdresses were bequeathed.

Crow Dog was the first to address us and get the service under way. He spoke of how it was good to see men wearing their hair long and also gave a long spiel about how one of Elmer's relatives had been the first to bring the sacred peyote into Rosebud. He talked about it for a long time, but I'm afraid most of his sun dancers couldn't see the point. Elmer had had nothing to do with grandfather peyote, as far as I know; he never even mentioned it. He also said something along the lines of, "Now you can go smoke that *pegi*," meaning now that Elmer was gone. He grinned as he said this and was looking right at me. Medicine men! Even

if you don't know 'em, you can't get a thing past 'em. Then the
drummers started warming up, and we all moved into the circle, coming in through the east gate and moving into our dance
places. I'd managed to borrow a whistle from a young man there,
and I was ready with it. Maybe a little too ready, for as the drums
and singers began, and we began dancing and moving about the
circle under the direction of Mr. Around Him, I began blowing
on mine, just as the others were doing. He was standing not far
from me, and something about it must have struck him as just
wrong, because I saw his head whip around toward me with his
mouth in a grimace of distaste. Just for a second, but I was more
careful with it after that.

We danced for a time, did the circle of the four directions,
and then came out and sat for a while on the grass, waiting for
the word to go up to the little hilltop, close to Irene's, where the
grave was. Gwen and I had talked the night before about how
nothing was being done according to Elmer's spoken wishes. He
hadn't wanted to be embalmed, but the family had gone ahead
and done it. He'd wanted to be buried over at a spot at the south-
eastern portion of his land, where, he said, at least one other
medicine man was buried. But the family was burying him at
the family plot, next to his late wife, Blanche. I found out from
Shannon, too, that soon after Gwen had been forced out, the boys
had moved in and had been using the Chev to run around par-
tying. Norman had just come in, demanded the keys, and taken
it. She also told me that when they were at the hospital and the
doctor had come in and told them that Elmer was gone, Gilli had
taken off immediately, gone back and broken into the school bus,
and stolen the suitcase. We sun dancers had tried, others besides
myself and Gwen, to shield him from his relatives—but at the
last, we couldn't.

It was strange. After the first time Gilli had come in with his
group to put up on the hill that spring, I couldn't get rid of the

notion that I had to shoot Gilli. I had a .50-caliber single- shot
black powder rifle in my camper, and I was almost ready to do
it. But when I went to open the breech, the mechanism jammed
shut! I tried everything to free it—three-in-one oil, solvent,
penetrating oil—but nothing would open it back up. It wasn't a
rational thought, just a powerful impulse. When I'd cooled down
enough to think it over, I realized I didn't want to be one more
white man shooting one more Indian. Plus, I didn't want to go to
prison; what would become of my little dogs? And my cat? Short
of that, however, there was no way to keep them from victimizing him. I'd also found out that Gilli wasn't one of Elmer's sons
at all. Blanche had been pregnant with him when she'd married
Elmer. He'd raised him as one of his own.

After the dance, the young man from whom I'd borrowed the
whistle came by for it, obviously anxious that it not "walk off."
I gladly returned it and thanked him for the use. Then it was
time for us all to get up and follow along after the hearse. Past
the sun-dance arbor, up the grassy hill, through some low trees
to the Running family plot. There were hundreds of people, some
in the sun by the grave, some shaded under the trees. I had never
walked this long way up to the very edge of Irene's property.
There was, of course, a high heap of earth next to the grave, with
the casket lying beside it.

I was so upset that I remember only a few details of the
burial. I recall Crow Dog speaking again, the women at the grave
singing in Lakota, and the casket being lowered down. Then the
family members and the senior sun-dance leaders, all male, got to
work backfilling with the shovels that were still there. I remember hanging back for a bit and having to take out my handker-
chief and hold it to my face as I began weeping again. Just as I
put it away, Mr. Around Him suddenly stepped up by my side. I
started back a bit, as he'd startled me. But he just stood right next
to me, not saying anything, and I got the feeling he was there

to lend friendly support. After a while, I got to where I felt like helping and took a turn or two with one of the shovels. Jason had been on the mound for a while already, throwing dirt with both hands, back in badger mode.

When it was all done, the time came for Crow Dog to distribute Elmer's eagle-feather war bonnets among his boys. He harangued them a bit, but I couldn't catch much of what was said. I just have a picture of Webster, Norman, and Gilli standing there with those headdresses on. It reminded me of the first time I saw Elmer in one of them, leading us dancers at Santee. He was so slight in his dancer's skirt and his head had been so hidden by the bonnet that it almost looked like there was nobody in there at all.

Then it was a weary trudge back. I'd bought new black boots, as well as a new black shirt and jeans, and they weren't even close to being broken in. They were hurting my feet, so I stopped and turned around after having gone a little way and stuck my thumb out at a passing car. This Indian fellow stopped right away, leaned over, and opened up the door. I thanked him for the ride, and we exchanged names. Turns out, he was a Leadercharge, just like the man I'd stopped for on the road to Rosebud and helped get gas for his stranded car. I almost asked him if he had a relative by the name of so-and-so, but I decided against it.

When we got back, there was a big feed waiting for everyone. Gwen, in a long dress, stood by a little table that was set up in the picnic area in front of the ceremony house. She talked about how Elmer had told her this day was coming, and so she'd baked these things for the sun dancers, in memory of Elmer, but she choked up and had to turn away.

I can no more remember much about the rest of the evening than I can the details of the graveside harangues; I was emotionally drained, nothing left. I recall on the way back to Mission, though, we stopped at the big, new organic foods supermarket that had just opened on the west edge of town. Gwen was getting a few things, and I stopped in the men's room. When I caught a look at myself in the mirror, I was shocked. I looked like hell warmed over, to put it mildly. I got some cold water on my face, and we went out, and I mentioned to Gwen that anyone could always tell if I was upset, it showed so strongly.

Anyway, later that evening, Gwen suddenly remembered something that had happened the day Grandpa died. She and I were sitting in the evening shade, in folding chairs outside her little trailer, when she sat bolt upright and said, "Karl, I've got to tell you about what happened. It was just about sunset the day Grandpa died. I didn't know anything was happening, but all of a sudden, this huge stream of dragonflies started flying right over my trailer! I was outside talking to Sharon, when there they were—thousands of them, going right overhead."

"Wow, that's amazing," I replied. "Did Elmer ever tell you what the teaching was about the dragonflies?"

"No!"

"He said, 'Them dragonflies, that's the warrior. They come in, do their business, and then they go.'"

"I wondered about them! They've come to me once or twice this last summer."

"Remember the second time there was a big moth on Grandpa's doorway?" I asked her. "The luna moth?"

"Uh-huh!"

"I remember seeing one then, just before sun dance. And then just afterward, a big dragonfly came flying past me. It was really close, and as it flew, it sort of made a little dip, right over the Chev pickup, right where I could see it. I had a feeling like that gift was being honored."

I maybe stayed on for another day or so, but it couldn't have been for long. My neighbors were taking care of the pups back home, and I had to get back.

*   *   *   *   *

MORE MEMORIES FROM THE EARLY DAYS AT THE OLD PLACE IN
Santee have come back, such as the time when I asked Patti about
the ban on having animals in the house. "The spirits can't get
past them if they're in your house with you," she said. Some
people might be praying for you, but all that would happen is
that you'd have healthy animals. Also, after we'd had the special
Indian tea at the end of ceremony, Elmer would always caution
the celebrants, "Don't touch them *sunkas* [dogs] right 'way."

And I recall Pete, at the new place, telling me about how if
even a bird strayed indoors, it had to be caught, and a *woluta*,
or red-felt tobacco tie, had to be tied to one of its legs, or else it
would fly away with the spirit of one of the occupants. "Patti
made me chase down this little bird," he told me, "and closed the
doors and windows until it was caught!"

Then there were the six-legged spiders that were always
showing up at Elmer's mobile home in Rosebud. And, the
moths—the lime-green luna moth and later the cecropia moth—
would be found clinging to the frame of the front door, early in
the morning, but sometimes later in the day too. There's an old
belief, way pre-Christian, that the souls of the departing take the
form of moths and butterflies. And those showed up just a few
weeks before his death.

Also, about the ceremony house—not only was the single
hundred-watt bulb unscrewed for every ceremony, but the door
was kept locked as well. Apparently, some years before my time,
ceremony had just gotten under way when someone opened the
door to get in, allowing the light from the security lamp in the
backyard to shine in.

At the old house in Santee, after a day's work on the new
one, just as dusk was beginning, a deer jumped across the road
right in front of me as I crossed a little bridge, so close I could
have counted the hairs on its rear right hock—no, the left one, it

was jumping right to left. I was so scared it was gonna come in through the windshield at me!

Or the evenings in Santee spent watching the basic-cable lineup on DirecTV after Elmer, Pete, and I had knocked off work for the day. All the while, I would wonder what in the hell this old-time Indian was making of the nutso commercials. Like for ladies' lingerie. It was hard to know what was going through his mind. I can sometimes get an idea of what another might be thinking through intuiting or observing, but not with the old man. The impression I got most of the time was that he just tolerated cable TV. Once a country-music news item caught his interest, though. First there was footage of the late singer, then the death announcement. Elmer asked, "Whozzat singer?"

"Hoyt Axton," replied one of the horseback riders.

Then there was the business with Elmer's personal food taboos. After the spirits called him and had given him his altar, he could no longer eat buffalo, since that was now one of his helping spirits. The thing with the little black-tailed deer was another matter. It seems, during his drinking days, he'd gone hunting with a rifle and killed a number of them. Later on, the deer spirit had spoken to him: "Why do you kill so many of my children? You already got enough to feed your family! From now on, when you eat that deer meat, you gon' be sick." He told us this at one of the sun dances in Santee, but by then, that deer was also one of his helpers.

Another thing I recall now is the matter of the old moonshiner. While we were first making the move to the new place in Santee, Patti was still being civil enough to tell us about it. It seems the old farm, and the old man on it, had a reputation on the Santee rez. "When I was a little girl," Patti told us, "that old man was the boogeyman. All us kids were scared to death of him. We used to dare each other to walk down here, but nobody did. Too scared."

A few weeks before I had to leave Santee that year, Elmer and I were working on the road. We came in for a break, and he said, "That ol' man used to live here, I hear him sometimes. He walks around in that basement, little bit, then he's quiet."

Talking of spirits, at one of the sun-dance meetings in Rosebud, the subject of ceremony ties came up. One fellow said, "Elmer, we have to change the sheet, the list of those ties. Add a blue one on the end because of that turtle that came to you."

Elmer just looked up and gave his assent. It seems that recently a little turtle had come and spoken to him, told him he was gonna be there and help out.

I've spoken with Gwen on the phone recently, and she again reminded me of a few things about Elmer. "Grandpa was about the woman."

She didn't elaborate on this, but as Gorgie remarked to me, "He always kept the men and women separate and in balance." Thinking about this myself, I realize how right they were.

He would never malign Patti, who ended up taking such advantage of him. The most he'd say was that she was crazy, but after a few months of being back in Rosebud, he told me he wasn't gonna say anything about her anymore. He was always polite to any female in his presence, and even after Irene and her brood had been terrorizing him for weeks and had taken his old sun-dance grounds away, he'd still sit and chat in Lakota with her when she chanced to stroll over for a visit. That's a good example.

At the beginning of my time in Rosebud in 2009, there was no doubt a male presence was needed out at Grandpa's. Besides the hassles from the relatives, there was a prowler hanging around. The rainy spell began shortly before I arrived, and during the first week, Gwen told me about how, one morning after a fall of rain, she'd gone outside to the front of the mobile home where the big kitchen windows were and found a man's boot tracks in the mud. Besides changing the locks on all the doors, including the ceremony house and getting the baby monitor for Elmer's bedroom, I also got a set of screw-in window locks.

As Gwen says, "Karl, we gave that old man a good last year. That's something we get to walk with for the rest of our lives." I just wish the other sun dancers would get it together to buy a headstone to mark the old man's grave. I will, eventually, if it has to be me, but with the sixth anniversary of his passing coming up, I miss him more and more and wish there was more I could do.

AFTERWORD I

Gwen's Dream

TWO OR THREE WEEKS AFTER THE FUNERAL, GWEN CALLED again. She'd called once or twice in the interim, mainly to complain about how the relatives at Elmer's mobile home were letting the place go to ruin and completely wasting the food in the garden. "What's wrong with them, Karl? Here they've got a garden full of food I put in, and they won't even harvest any of it! They just go into town and eat that fast-food shit!"

I'd also had a call from Norman's wife, Shannon, asking me whether I'd gotten the new furniture for Elmer or for Gwen! Seems Gwen had taken some of the nicer pieces I'd bought and moved them into storage. I wanted to say to Shannon, "Hey, greedy, your father-in-law just passed away, the oldest *wicasa wakan* your people had, and you're hassling about the furniture?!"

But I didn't. I told her I'd gotten the furniture for whoever was at the trailer with Grandpa to use. It was for him and the people who did for him.

"Oh," she said.

But another call came from Gwen one afternoon. She sounded a bit flustered as she told me, "Karl, I have to tell you about this dream I had last night. I went to bed and I was praying to

Tunkasila, asking him how we got from Elmer being there to his being gone so fast. And I dreamed he was back in his bedroom, lying there, and Gilli was in there, yelling at him to give him some money, and Grandpa said, 'No, goddamn it! No more money!' And Gilli hauled off and hit him."

I learned later from another source that at the hospital, they'd removed big chunks of food from Elmer's airway.

Personally, I believe Gwen's dream. It's consistent with Gilli's behavior, and it explains why he stayed as far away as possible from me at the funeral.

So, the heart-attack story given out by the family is not true, at least for me.

AFTERWORD II

My Dream

EARLY IN THE WINTER OF 2009, I HAD A DREAM OF MY OWN. Not to toot my own horn, but Gwen and Sage had been left with almost no resources, after having been kicked to the curb by the relatives, a description Gwen was generous enough to include me in as well—meaning they'd done the same to me. I'd been sending Sage and Gwen some help—care packages, mostly flour and baking supplies for her home business, and comic books and stuff for Sage, since I knew he liked them. Gwen's job in Mission hadn't panned out, and they had moved to a small suburb of Rapid City. I only mention that I helped out with this, because I know the grandfathers are always watching, and I like to think I merited some help of my own.

But one night, I dreamed that Elmer and I were riding in a pickup truck, not the Chev, but the old Ford he'd had in Santee. We were going down a dirt road, and at first it seemed that I was driving, and he was sitting in the passenger's seat, then that he was driving. Next, we were sitting together, outside, on the edge of a flat-roofed, brick building. Wherever this was, it felt like the last building on the edge of town. There was a big woods spread out beneath us. Next, we were still sitting together, but the rooftop had changed into a high sandstone ledge, the same yellow color that the bricks of the building had been. We were much higher up than before, and there was nothing but blue sky above and the green forest below. I was holding a long buckskin bag, like a pipe bag but undecorated and tied with a twist of rawhide at the open end. Elmer took it and began pulling out all this unpleasant-looking stuff, like rotten feathers. As his hand got deeper in, I could see something in there was moving on its own! He reached and drew out this strange, quivering clawlike thing. It was like two eagle quills together, coming to a point and dark yellow and green. Altogether, it looked about six inches long, darkening to black at the blunt end. He held it between his first and second fingers, looked me right in the eye, and, without speaking, just flipped it away.

I woke up immediately, really excited. Since I first started praying in the Indian way, back in 1986, I'd had other dreams into which Native men had come. There's a profound difference between this dream and the usual ones. One is just the human mind, asleep, sorting out the day's, the life's, events. The other is a real communication.

AFTERWORD III

The Trial

SOMETIME LATE IN THE WINTER OF 2010, FEBRUARY OR March, I received a phone call from Lorna. She told me Norman was to attend a hearing in Rapid City the next week. Seems there was some question concerning the title he'd presented to the county clerk—a question about him being named the owner of the Chev. She told me the judge wanted me to testify by telephone, and she gave me a number to call as well as a numerical code that would get me connected to the hearing. She was very peremptory in her tone, I must say—pretty much telling me what to do and when to do it, without bothering with any pleases or thank-yous. I made it until almost the end of the conversation before a little growl began to creep into my voice. Then she remembered her manners.

Anyway, the first thing I did was to call Gwen and tell her the time of the hearing. She already knew the place. I also gave her the code, since I figured they wouldn't let her in without authorization. (No one told me not to share it!) She said she'd be there, sounded keenly interested, even eager. So when Lorna called back, just to confirm the exact time, I said I'd call in, for sure. And thanks!

Well, the appointed time rolled around, and I called in to the courthouse in Rapid City and gave my code on the automated prompt. I was immediately on speakerphone in the courtroom. The judge introduced himself and told me to wait a little, until someone else also called in. Gwen told me later that Gilli had shown up, with his better half, and he looked "like he'd been run over." I imagine he also wanted the pickup. Then after I said, "Hello, Your Honor," he swore me in.

The judge started questioning Norman. It seems the title he had with his name on it had been presented in copy form, not as the original. Shannon's name was on it too, and he testified several times that she had done the paperwork on the truck. The judge started asking him if she was not present to testify, and he said she wasn't, adding, "I wish she was." Then it was my turn.

I was asked when I'd given the pickup to Elmer.

"In the spring of 2009, Your Honor."

Then a lot of questions from him, including whether it had been an exchange or a sale.

"No, it was a gift."

Then more questions as to the time and circumstances, and finally, when I'd purchased the pickup myself.

I'd been asked by Lorna to get a copy of the bill of sale from the dealership and send it to the court. So the judge had that in front of him when he asked Norman, "Mr. Running, when did your father give this truck to you?"

"In 2008, Your Honor, when he was alive."

"Of course he did it when he was alive!" stormed the judge. Next, he asked Norman if he understood the penalties for perjury. Then asked a few more of me, ending with, "Is there any way that Elmer Running could have come into possession of this vehicle in 2008, a year before you bought it and gave it to him?"

"In no way, Your Honor."

At about that point, the hearing was adjourned, and I couldn't help feeling sorry, a little, for Norman. It was so pathetic; he'd sounded like a little boy caught with his hand in the cookie jar. At the last, I could hear Gwen asking the judge about the pickup Elmer had given her and the judge politely replying that there wasn't anything he could do about it. A year or so later, the FBI came into Rosebud and arrested Shannon for mail fraud.

In 2010, Gorgie and Lorna and some others decided to begin holding memorial sun dances for Grandpa. There was a hope that the ceremony the old man had worked so hard to bring about not simply come to an end. Unfortunately, I couldn't attend the first one. I had gotten involved with a woman in Minnesota, where I had a little summer shack, and the romance quickly devolved into a series of legal and financial obligations—or at least what I thought were obligations on my part. Things didn't work out between us in a big way, but they did keep me occupied most of the summer.

There was another memorial the next August. I was back in Minnesota, on my own, and I recall being on the phone with Gorgie and telling her I wouldn't be able to attend because I was having a hip replaced in September. My right one had gotten so bad, I had to use a cane indoors and out. It would go out from under me without notice. "That's a good reason for not dancing," she replied.

The third year, 2012, I stayed in Nebraska all summer. I was still in touch with Gwen but was too worn out with everything I'd undergone the previous two years. Gwen called me after the first week in August. "Karl, you're not gonna believe what happened at sun dance this year!" she began. "They were having the third memorial dance, went through the four days of purification, but on the fourth day, when the tree went up, no sooner had they put it up and gotten it set, then this gust of wind comes outta nowhere from the west, pulls the tree up, and lays it down toward the east gate, without so much as breaking a branch or taking off a leaf! Gorgie called me and told me about it. They had a *wicasa wakan* there, Roy Stone, and he went into the sweat lodge and came back with, 'That Elmer was the one that did it. He said, 'No more sun dance. He's busy looking after his relatives, there on the other side.'"

During the years since Elmer's walking on, some other sun dances have sprung up, or tried to. Norman set up a sun-dance grounds, but I've heard nothing about how it went. The year after the funeral, I was in touch with Dino. I wasn't quite giving full credence to Gwen's assessment of him, and he'd asked me if I still had the drum I'd brought in 2008. We got to talking one time, and I sort of agreed I'd give his sun dance a try. I even bought a few shovels and some skulls, but when I told Gwen about it, she asked, "What do you want to do that for?" She reminded me of how Dino and his clique had behaved in 2009 and how he'd brought Vern Yellowhawk back after Vern had ripped off Grandpa and played me for a chump—not to mention Grandpa had struck Vern with his cane and declared he didn't want him around. Dino also told me he'd set up an arbor the year before, but someone on the rez had come in and "cut down the uprights for firewood." That got me thinking, maybe it wasn't done for firewood, and I abandoned the idea.

Gwen recently reminded me that Norman didn't go to jail, but Shannon did. Seems she was soliciting funds from people to "take care of Grandpa" after he'd passed on.

I guess Gilli's still running his sun dance, and a few of Elmer's dancers go there. It reminds me of what Elmer told me one day in early summer of 2000: "Gilli's gon' be a medicine man." That's all he said. The spirits must have told it him, but he seemed mystified by it. Later on, sometime around 2006 or 2007, I was told, Gwen said he'd banned Gilli and Iktomi from his sun dance—essentially saying they were unfit to dance anymore. Gilli had been drunk, and he showed up at Elmer's when Norman and Webster were there and knifed them. The disqualifying factor wasn't the drunkenness; it was the shedding of a relative's blood. "That's the rules—from Sitting Bull!" Elmer had once exclaimed to me on another matter, but yet pertaining to the sun dance.

Al Running, Elmer's brother, has been overseeing Gilli's sun dance to see that things are done right, but I still won't attend, not after hearing Gwen's dream. At the disposal of Elmer's ceremonial possessions, Crow Dog had decreed that each of his sons was to have the suitcase containing the altar for one year apiece. But when it came time for Gilli to give it up to whoever was next, he wouldn't do it. He held on to it for months, until finally Crow Dog went out to Gilli's place himself to demand it. Only the worst kind of fool would defy a medicine man in such a matter, and Gilli's *win* was smarter than he was. She grabbed the suitcase and ran out and gave it to Leonard.

Once, when we were talking about other people copying Elmer's monthly ceremony—specifically, the Englishwoman who ran the White Horse Trading Post in Mission and her Lakota husband—Elmer had said to me, "Monkey see, monkey do; that's the way the monkey learns."

Gwen and I have a saying between us: "What's so hard to understand about 'No more sun dance'?" I realize how hard it may be to give up participation. If done correctly, it's real magic; it really is "the power to make things grow" (*wakan*). But to quote one of Black Elk's granddaughters, "There are people all over the earth who are suffering because the sun dance is not being done in the right way."

It puts me in mind of a news flash Elmer and Patti had gotten about one of their lady dancers when we were all back at the old place in Santee. I may be confusing two accounts, but at one time Elmer was doing the *hunka*, or "making of relatives" ceremony. One white lady was so honored and went home and let the perceived status go completely to her head. She once took another woman's pipe away because the cloth squares she was using for prayer ties weren't exactly one inch square! When Elmer heard about it, he shouted, "That's bullshit!" And the woman who was throwing her weight around like that, her husband had a heart attack not long afterward.

Once, Elmer and I were working on the yard at Santee, I can't recall if it was before or after sun dance, but these two older boys showed up one day around noon and relayed a request for Elmer to come sing a little at someone else's sun dance on the Santee rez. Elmer spoke to them for a spell in Lakota, then turned to me. "I told those boys they shoulda brought me a pipe or at least a little tobacco!" When they arrived at this dance, we'd brought his drum and got there near the end of a dance round. The leader got up and talked about the dancers' dedication, considering how hot it was. But Elmer noticed that whoever was in charge was letting the dancers smoke and drink coffee during the rest breaks. Elmer spoke then, in Lakota, and may have sung a song or two. But as we left, he turned to me and said, "You seen them dancers? Smokin', drinkin' coffee? 'Cause o' that, they could dance all day, no rests, but they still wouldn't see nothing out of it!"

Now, as I've said, some of the sun dancers are going to Norman's sun dance or some to Florian Bluethunder's, and some even go to Gilli's. Some go on to the dances at Pine Ridge or elsewhere after dancing at Rosebud. Gwen and I talk regularly and share what we remember of what Grandpa was and what he said to us. Gwen reminded me he always warned us not to go to other sun dances.

"Once, this woman called for Elmer," Gwen told me. "She said she had cancer and was asking Elmer to pray for her. I told him, and he said, 'I told the people, no animals in the house. She had a cat.' And he said it so matter-of-factly," she finished.

So now, even if I felt like it, I don't know where I'd go to dance or even sweat. Almost none of the old-timers are left— old-timers who know the old ways and the old rules, and who, as Gorgie said of Grandpa, keep the men and women separate and in balance with each other. I tried to start sweating with a Dakota man in Nebraska a few years back, but he had the men and women together, and it felt just too wrong after I tried it once. I even felt a little sick afterward.

It is now six years since Elmer's death, or perhaps I should say murder. Everyone wants to do something, but no one seems to know what. A while after Gwen had told me of her dream, we were discussing it, and I said, "Gwen, if it's true, then he died just as Sitting Bull and Crazy Horse did—at the hands of his own people."

I know that writing all this unvarnished stuff may not win me any friends. I hope the Indian people don't take it as just another book by some *wasicu* about how bad we are. I have written it simply because my old college roommate encouraged me to write a book about "all the wild people you've met." Also, because of the encouragement offered by Elmer's brother, Al: "It's good you wrote something about my brother." Of course, I haven't put in everything! That would be too long and tedious a read for anyone. But I still feel apprehensive I've left out something important or maybe said too much.

This is simply a memoir, written from memory—with all the lapses and lacunae and distortions that implies—about the best man I ever met.

Afterword IV

The Outer-Space People

I'VE RESISTED WRITING THIS CHAPTER—AND PUTTING ITS CON-
tents in their proper place in the sequence of events—for fear
that it'd get the entire book dismissed as "kook" literature. But
Elmer claimed to be a contactee. It was while we were still at the
old house in Santee one evening. It was during that brief interval
after Pete had taken off for his spree and before the flood that ru-
ined the well and almost canceled sun dance. Patti wasn't around;
most nights that was the case. She was off gambling at the casino.
"Going to work," as she put it. Elmer and I'd been working on
the grounds as usual, we'd had the evening meal, and we were
just sitting around, smoking and talking.

Our conversation drifted around to the pipe, and I mentioned
to him that I'd heard that the original *canunpa*, given to the
people by the White Buffalo Calf Woman, was no longer in the
keeping of the Looking Horse family out west as was generally
supposed, but had been spirited away and sold to a collector.
Elmer said nothing directly to this but began telling a story of
how, a few years back, an Indian man had come by and either
gifted him or tried to sell him some eagle feathers. Probably a gift
or trade was made, for I can't believe Grandpa would buy them

with money. Either way, he ended up with them and said, "Them feathers was real old. That night I couldn't get to sleep!"

My memory of the conversation's a little hazy at this point, but it seemed that this was somehow connected with what he said next. It seems there'd been another night when he was alone in the little farmhouse, and he'd been awakened in the middle of the night by a bright light shining in through the window. "I don' care if you believe me or not, but it was the outer-space people." I was so taken aback by this, I couldn't attend to what he said next—something about their offering him a helmet, or a piece of some kind of equipment that would allow him to come aboard their ship. I believe a silvery suit of some kind was also mentioned, but he said that, when they offered to take him on board, he declined, frankly admitting he was too much afraid, and who wouldn't be? There was little drama in his recounting of this, and the matter-of-fact way he told me about the incident only served to freak me out even more.

I've always held to the Nebraska naturalist Loren Eiseley's explanation of why there are no (open) alien visitations: for the same reasons that we can't travel to other planets. The distances and the time needed to traverse them are simply too great. This was going through my head as he was speaking, making me miss even more.

But he didn't have too much more to say about it then. It came up a few more times later on. We were again alone together at the mobile home in Rosebud in late 2000, and we were talking about how the planet, the Mother Earth, was in a bad way. He brought up the potential destruction of a meteor strike of vast proportions. Except he confused the term *meteor*, with *comet*. "That comet," he'd said, "that could come most any time. We gotta pray with our pipes, ask that comet to keep 'way from us."

I mentioned to him that, at a recent new moon, I'd gotten my *canunpa* down and done just that.

"I been tellin' the people," he replied.

"Elmer," I said, "if it did hit, would there be any people left alive?"

He looked solemnly at me from under his brows. "Just a few," he replied, almost in a whisper.

And once again, in 2008, during one of the winter months after Gwen and Sage had come back but before Elmer'd had his second stroke, Gwen was on the phone with one of the longtime sun dancers. I believe it was Sage who called her attention to the strange lights moving around in the sky. It was such a bizarre occurrence that Gwen left the phone on the kitchen table off the hook and called, "Grandpa! You've got to come and see this!" Well, he roused himself out of the back bedroom and was down the hall on his cane pretty quick, but when he looked out the door for himself, he was unimpressed. "It's just the outer-space people!" he exclaimed and stumped on back. The person on the other end of the line heard all this and was laughing hard when Gwen picked up the receiver. I still don't know what to think. I've never seen one, so I can't really have an opinion.

I seem to recall that he brought them up once more, when he was living back in Rosebud during the winter of 2000/01. It was the evening after I'd mentioned that I'd followed his advice about praying to avert "that comet." He said the outer-space people had told him that people who were following the traditional Indian way, when they crossed over, they'd go to the happy hunting grounds. Christians would go to heaven when they died, and the people who'd come to pray with him would go to be with him when they walked on. I wish I could recall his exact language in this, but that was the sense of it. I did not disbelieve it. "First, we're on this side, then we go to the other side."

Resources

Oyate Owanjila

THIS DIGITAL RECORDING WAS MADE ON NOVEMBER 25, 1995, in the ceremony house of Norbert Elmer Running and Patti Running.

The singers are Elmer Running, a Lakota spirit interpreter, and Patti Running's sons, Leo Chinana and Jamie Chinana.

The producer, such as I am, along with many who have the good fortune of knowing them, wish to thank Elmer and Patti for the continued openness, guidance, and help we have received, both for our families and ourselves. You have helped so many and open your doors to all those who look for a deeper understanding of this walk we all travel on our Holy Grandmother Earth. As for myself, I have so much more to learn...

Thanks to Robert Jennik, a fellow traveler, for planting the seeds for this project.

Wakantan hot anin yelo! Pilamaya pelo!
—David W. Ross

Coyote Song

Kola miye ca he wa u welo
Kola miye ca he wa u welo
Wamayanka yo wa u welo
Canunpa wan uha wa u welo
Kola miye ca he wa u welo
Wamayanka yo wa u welo
Wakan nawajin miye ca he wa u welo
Kola miye ca he wa u welo
Wamayanka yo wa u welo
Hoye wi ki iyoklata ya he
Wociciyakin kta ca he wa u welo
Wamayanka yo wa u welo
Anpo wichacpi ki iyoklata ya he
Wociciyakin kta ca he wau welo
Wamayanka yo wa u welo
Anpo wi ki iyoklata ya he
Wociciyakin kta ca he wa ti welo
Wamayanka yo wa u welo

Friend, it is me who is coming
Friend, it is me who is coming
Look at me, I am coming
With a Pipe I am coming
Friend, it is me who is coming
Look at me, I am coming
Standing sacredly, I am coming
Friend, it is me who is coming
Look at me, I am coming
Under the Moon
I am coming to talk to you

Look at me, I am coming
Under the Stars
I am coming to talk to you
Look at me, I am coming
Under the Sun
I am coming to talk to you
Look at me, I am coming

Pipe-Filling Song

Kola lecel ecun wo
Kola lecel ecun wo
Kola lecel ecun wo
Hecanu ki, ni Tunkasila
waniyang u ktelo

Friend, do it in this manner
Friend, do it in this manner
Friend, do it in this manner
Do this and your Grandfather
will come to see you

Canunpa wanji y uha ilotake ci
miksuya opagi yo
Hecanu ki, taku yacin ki
iyece tu ktelo

Kola lecel ecun wo
Kola lecel ecun wo
Kola lecel ecun wo
Hecantt ki, ni Tunkasila
waniyang, u ktelo

Hochoka wanji, yuha ilotake ci

miksuya opagi yo
Hecanu ki, taku yacin ki
iyece tu ktelo

When you begin with the Pipe
remember me as you fill it
Do this, and whatever you desire
will come true

Friend, do it in this manner
Friend, do it in this manner
Friend, do it in this manner
Do this and your Grandfather
will come to see you

When you begin this sacred ritual,
remember me as you fill the Pipe
Do this, and whatever you desire
will come true

Four Directions Song

Wiocpayata etuwan yo
Ni Tukasila ahituwan yankelo
Cekiya yo, cekiya yo!
Ahituwan yankelo
Waziyalakiya duwan yo
Ni Tukasila ahil'u wan yankelo
Cekiya yo, cekiya yo! Ahituwan yankelo
Wiohiyanpata etuwan yo
Ni Tukasila ahituwan yankelo
Cekiya yo, cekiya yo! Ahituwan yankelo
Itokagata ahituwan yo

Ni Tukasila ahituwan yankelo
Cekiya yo, cekiya yo! Ahituwan yankelo
Wakatankiya ahituwan yo
Wakan Tanka heciye he yankelo
Cekiya yo, cekiya yo! Ahituwan yankelo
Makatakia ahituwan yo
Unsi Maka kin heciye he yunkelo
Cekiya yo, cekiya yo! Ahituwan yunkelo

Look to the West
Your Grandfather sits there looking this way
Pray, pray! He sits there looking this way
Look to the North
Your Grandfather sits there looking this way
Pray, pray! He sits there looking this way
Look to the East
Your Grandfather sits there looking this way
Pray, pray! He sits there looking this way
Look to the South
Your Grandfather sits there looking this way
Pray, pray! He sits there looking this way
Look to the Sky
The Great Spirit sits there waiting for you
Pray, pray! He sits there looking this way
Look to the Earth
Grandmother Earth lies there waiting for you
Pray, pray! She lies there looking this way

Prayer / Sweat-Lodge Song

Tunkasila iwankiyo
Tunkasila iwankiyo
Tunkasila iwankiyo
Ikce wicasa yakun le miye yelo

Wiohpeyata oyate wan waniyang u ktelo
Hocoka wan ociciya yelo
Ikce wicasa yakun le miye yelo

Grandfather, take a close look
Grandfather, take a close look
Grandfather, take a close look
The People, this is us
To the West a nation is coming to see you
A sacred center, I have told you
The People, this is us

Prayer Song

Wakan Tanka tokaheya cewaki yelo
Wakan Tanka tokaheya cewaki yelo
mitakuye ob wani kta ca hoye wa yelo
Tunkasila, toka heya.

I pray to the Great Spirit first
I pray to the Great Spirit first
I want to live with my relatives, I send a voice
I pray to the Great Spirit first
I want to live with my relatives, I send a voice
I pray to my Grandfather first
I want to live with my relatives, I send a voice

Spirit-Calling Song

Kola le miye ca wa u welo
Kola le miye ca wa u welo, wa u welo
Kola le miye ca wa u welo, wa u welo
Wiocpeyata
I nawajiin na ahituwan nawajin yelo

Kola le miye ca wa u welo, wa u welo

Friend, this is me, I am coming
Friend, this is me, I am coming, I am coming
Friend, this is me, I am coming, I am coming
To the West
I am standing here and looking toward you
Friend, this is me, l am coming, I am coming

Prayer Song

Wakan Tanka unsimala yo
He makakijelo
Canunpa kile he uha hoye wa yelo
Wakan Tanka unsimala yo
He makakiyelo
Canunpa kile he uha hoye wa yelo

Great Spirit, have pity on me
as I am suffering
Holding this Pipe, I am sending a voice
Great Spirit, have pity on me
as I am suffering
Holding this Pipe, I am sending a voice

Prayer Song

Tunkasila Wakan Tanka heya hoye wa yelo
Tunkasila Wakan Tanka heya hoye wa yelo
Tunkasila omakiyayo makakijelo

Grandfather, Great Spirit, I am sending a voice
Grandfather, Great Spirit, I am sending a voice
Grandfather, help me, as I am suffering

Prayer Song
Vocables

Medicine Song

Pejuta wan cicu kta ca
Wayankiye yo

I will give you a medicine
Look this way!

Stone Song

Hokaowin u welo
Hokaowin u welo
Iyanwan wakanyan yunkina wana,
Hokaowin u welo
Hokaowin u welo wakanyan u welo

It is coming around
It is coming around
Now a stone in a sacred manner
Is coming around
Is coming around in a sacred manner

Spider Song

Kola wayanki yo!
Iktomi oyate wan waniyang u welo
Siyo tanka hot anin waciyang u welo

Friend, look!
A spider nation comes to see you
Blowing an Eagle-Bone Whistle, they come dancing

Spider Song

Cokala wakan u mica kaga kta ca
Cokata eya ya nawajin yelo
Kola le ehek'un lecun welo

He shall prepare a sacred center for me
Standing in the center, I send a voice
Friend, you have said, do it in this manner

Prayer Song

Tunkasila wamayank u yo
Tunkasila wamayank u ye yo
Tunkasila wamayank u ye yo
Ikce wicasa Tacanunpi wan yuha hoye wa yelo
Mitakuye ob wani kta ca, eyaya hoye wa yelo

Grandfather, look at me
Grandfather, look at me
Grandfather, look at me
Holding the People's Pipe, I am sending a voice
I send a voice saying, "I shall live with my relatives"

Pipe Song

Hoyeya yo, Hoyeya yo! Hoyeya yo, Hoyeya yo!
Tunkasila, leun kelo
Ikce wicasa Tacanunpi kin
Le yuha hoyeya yo
Hoyeya yo
Tunkasila, leun kelo

I beseech you, I beseech you!
I beseech you, I beseech you!

Grandfather, you have said
"The People's Pipe
Cry out with it"
I beseech you!
Grandfather, you have said

Offering Song

Lenake wayang u ye yo
Lenake wayang u ye yo
Waunye kin lena hoye miciciya yo
He mitakuye ob waniya waon wacin yelo
Tunkasila omakiya yo
Canli pahta kin lena hoye micidya yo
He mitakuye ob zaniya waon wacin yelo,
Tunkasila omakiya yo

Behold these that I have offered you
Behold these that I have offered you
I have pledged myself with this cloth
I shall live in good health with my relatives
Grandfather, help me!
I have pledged myself with these prayer ties
I shall live in good health with my relatives
Grandfather, help me!

Offering Song

Tunkan, unsi unlapi ye yo
Tunkan, unsi unlapi ye yo
He mitakuye ob wani kta ca
Lena cicu welo

Stone Spirits, have pity on us
Stone Spirits, have pity on us

I shall live with my relatives
I give you these offerings

Offering Song

Hoye tani nyan kin najin pelo
Hoye tani nyan kin najin pelo
Tunkasila la wokonze ca
Lena cicu welo

Our voices are heard as we leave
Our voices are heard as we leave
It is Grandfather's will
That I give you these offerings

Offering Song

Kola lena cicu welo, wayankiye yo
Kola lena cicu welo, wayankiye yo
Anpetu okihica cicu welo, wayankiye yo

Friend, these I have offered you. Behold them!
Friend, these I have offered you. Behold them!
The day has made it possible to make an offering
Behold them!

Thunder Being Song

Leciya ya tuwan maki pan pelo
Leciya ya tu wan maki pan pelo
Wiocpeyata wakinyan oyate wan
Kola maki pan pelo
Leciya ya tuwan maki pan pelo

Wiocpeyata wakinyan oyale wan
Kola maki pan pelo

Over here they are calling for me
Over here they are calling for me
To the West is a Thunder Being nation
My friends are calling for me
Over here they are calling for me
To the West is a Thunder Being nation
My friends are calling for me

SIDE B

Four Directions Song

Wiocpeyatakiya etuwan yo
Ni Tunkashila ahituwan yankelo
Cekiya yo, cekiya yo! Ni zani ktelo

Waziyatakiya etuwan yo
Canunpa wan ahituwan yankelo
Cekiya yo, cekiya yo! Ni zani ktelo

Wiohiyanpatakiya etuwan yo
Ni Tukasila ahituwan naji yelo
Cekiya yo, cekiya yo! Ni zani ktelo

Itokagatatakiya etuwan yo
Akatusni wa waniyang uktelo
Cekiya yo, cekiya yo! Ni zani ktelo

Look to the West
Your Grandfather sits there looking this way
Pray, pray! You shall have good health

Look to the North
A Pipe sits there looking this way
Pray, pray! You shall have good health

Look to the East
Your Grandfather stands there looking this way
Pray, pray! You shall have good health

Look to the South
A ghost is coming to see you
Pray, Pray! You shall have good health

Stone Song

Hoyemakiya yo, Cemakiye yo
Taku yacinki iyece tu ktelo
Tunkan sabicya eya
ca hoye waki yelo
Cemakiya yo, Hoye makiya yo
Taku yacinki iyece tu ktelo
Tunkan sabicya eya
ca hoye waki yelo

Send a voice to me, pray to me!
Whatever you want will be given
A blackened stone, you have said
so I send a voice to you
Pray to me, send a voice to me!
Whatever you want will be given
A blackened stone, you have said
so I send a voice to you

Spider Song

Maka sitomniyan
Okiya wa u welo
Iktomi wan heyaya u welo
Miye mawakan yelo

Throughout the world
I come to help
A spider says this as he comes
Me, I am sacred

Spider Song

Cannunpa wani ca u pelo
Tanyan yuzo yo
Ognas mayagna yecilo
Hena wakanyan iwa yelo
Ognas mayagna yecilo
Iktomi zi iceya miye yelo
Taku aiwayeci hena wakanyan
Iwa yelo
Ognas mayagna yecilo

You live through this Pipe
Hold it in a good way!
Maybe you will try to fool me
The things that I say are sacred
Maybe you will try to fool me
I am the yellow spider
The things that I say are sacred
Maybe you will try to fool me

Sundance Songs

Entrance Song
Vocables

Prayer Song

Tunkasila wamayanki yo
Le miye ca teciya nawanjielo
Unci maka naweci cena
 Wowakwala wa uha wau welo

Grandfather, look at me
Grandfather, look at me
This is me standing here, having a difficult time
I stand up for Mother Earth
I come in a humble manner

Prayer Song

Tunkasila, hoye wayinkta, namak'un yeyo
Maka sitomniyan, hoye wanikte, namak'un yeyo
Mitakuye ob wani ktelo
Cewelo

Grandfather, I am going to pray, hear me!
To the Universe, I am going to pray, hear me!
I shall live with my relatives
I am praying

Prayer Song
Vocables

Pipe Song

Canunpa wan uha hoye wa yelo
Oyate kin yanipi kta ca
Lecamu welo
Tunkasila, omakiya yo, omakiya yo

I'm sending a voice with this Pipe!
So that the people will live
I am doing this
Grandfather, help me, help me

Prayer Song

Wicasila wan tewahila k'un
Wan weglakin kta hunse

There was a man that I loved so dearly
Yes, I shall see my man again

Pipe Song

Oyate, wamayanka po!
Oyate, wamayanka po!
Canunpa wakan ca yuha cewaki yelo
Oyate, yanipi kta ca
Lecamu welo

People, look at me! People, look at me!
This Pipe I hold and pray with is sacred
People, you shall live
That is why I do this

Thanksgiving Song

Tunkasila
pilamaya ye, pilimaya ye, pilamaya yelo
Wicozzani wamayan k'un ca
pilamaya yelo

Grandfather,
I give thanks, I give thanks, I give thanks
You said you will help
I see good health, so
I give thanks, I give thanks

Tobacco Ties for Ceremonies

The following instructions are for the altar of Elmer Norbert Running, a Lakota interpreter.

SPIDER SPIRIT'S ALTAR

2 black (West) black horse
1 red (North) buffalo
1 yellow (East) all animals and spirits of the dead

ALTAR TIES FOR HELPING AND THANKS CEREMONIES

2 white (South) black-tailed deer and holy road
1 blue (Sky) creator
1 green (Earth) grandmother
1 red felt for the people
100: 25 each of yellow, blue, green, and white (all spirits, for doctoring and help)
75: 37 red and 38 yellow (or vice versa) (spirits who watch outside—these evaluate spirits that want to enter the ceremony and sends bad spirits away)
24: red (for help)
12: 6 blue and 6 green (spotted eagle)
24: white (holy road)
6: 3 blue and 3 green (spotted eagle)
6: all white (white spider)
5: all black (spider that paints himself black)
2: 1 black and 1 white (thunder clowns)
2: 1 black and 1 red (walks in the light)
4: 1 each of black, red, yellow, and white (Stone Nation)
4: 1 each of yellow, blue, green, and white (black-tailed deer)
2: 1 blue and 1 black (Fox "Walks Slow" Han Heya Man)
1: 1 blue (Turtle Tokala)

7: 1 each, in order: black, red, yellow, white, green, blue, small red felt (Ishnala Man, "Walks Alone)

2: 1 each of green and red (Wishasha Spring Water Man)

4: 1 each of yellow, black, red, blue

8: 6 green (*pejutayankan*) and 2 green with cormeal (buffalo)

24: blue

6: 1 red tie on 6 individual strings, six inches long (each goes on a different flag pole)

HEALING TIES (ADD TO THE ABOVE)

100 each of black, red, yellow, and white—or green, blue, yellow, and white. Add 5 black ties at the end (thunder clown altar)

FOR DOCTORING AND FOR HELP:

For spotted eagle:

24 bags (12 black, 12 white)

Flags: 1 each of black, white, blue, and green

12 bags (6 black, 6 white)

24 bags (12 blue, 12 green) for healing

12 bags (6 blue, 6 green) for help

BLACK STONE (STONE MESSENGER) ALTAR

Altar: 104 ties, 100 red and 1 tie each of black, red, yellow, and white

6: all red individual ties

6: 3 blue, 3 green (for spotted eagle)

FLAGS:

1 each of black, red, yellow, white, and red felt

TIES FOR A VISION QUEST

All of the Spider Spirits altar ties, plus:

100 each in the following order—green, blue, white, yellow, red, and black. Leave about one inch between each tobacco bag. These will be used to enclose the space where you stay on the hill.

1 yard each—black, red, yellow, white, blue, green, and red felt.

Abalone shell, fresh eagle feather, blanket, knife, bucket and dipper (optional)

FOR HELP WITH EMERGENCY OR SERIOUS SITUATION:

50 red ties on one string

More Detailed Information and Explanations

Elmer Running warns people not to put themselves above the pipe. He also does not have much understanding of the word *traditional* or sun dances that are "Indian only," as he says there are almost no true 100 percent Lakotas, and now almost all Indians from Pine Ridge and Rosebud (where his relatives come from) are "mixed-bloods" who are Sioux. These are English-speaking descendants of the original seven bands of the great Sioux Nation. Although never conquered by the Europeans (Elmer proudly displays the American flag, representing the one taken from the Seventh Cavalry at Little Big Horn), reservations were meant to destroy Lakota traditions, religious beliefs, language, and family bonds. Very few of the original ceremonies can be gotten from books or people. Only those who commune with the spirits know how modern-day people can follow the Lakota way of life. Elmer is a human, but if asked in the appropriate way (you need not offer him tobacco for every question you have at the sun dance), he can explain what is tradition, what was told to him by medicine men and interpreters, and what is told to him by the spirits since he received his vision and his altar more than twenty years ago.

Elmer believes that people have one mind and one heart—their own. He will rarely say no if asked by someone if what they want to do is OK. His English is not very good, but his wife, Patti, has an excellent command of English and will tell you what the spirits have told Elmer, what is Elmer's personal opinion, and what is her own personal opinion. She can assist you in asking a question in a way to find out if the answer is one that the spirits have or will tell to Elmer when he is acting as an interpreter. He was told that he was to be an interpreter by the spirits and not a medicine man. He is recognized as a medicine man by many, but he insists that a medicine man knows how to use herbs, salves, and potions to cure illnesses and ailments. In his ceremonies, the spirits do all the healing, under the watchful eye of Wakan Takan. He performs both *lowampi* and *yuwipi* ceremonies for healing, as well as leading the annual All Nations Sun Dance. At times, the spirits do tell him to use certain things to help heal people, so in this he is like a medicine man. The spirits who work through him are very powerful and not only protect him but have cured many seriously ill people. In all the ceremonies, people should make prayer ties, and Patti can tell people which combinations of colors and numbers are required for each ceremony. Men and women are separate during any of the sacred Lakota ceremonies. The spirits use the prayer ties, and they are important for the people to make before, during, or after a ceremony.

There are not firm rules or regulations (although this document may seem like that to some), as people have become used to in the white man's society, but there are definitely right and wrong things to do around the altar. You will hear people talk of "respect." All things are based upon this concept of respect to others, the pipe, the spirits, and Wakan Takan. In the end, the only punishment that people will likely receive is a stern comment from sun dancers or the security people, being made fun of by the sun dancers if the first comment is ignored, and finally the spirits themselves may intercede. Elmer rarely kicks out anyone for what they do on the sun-dance grounds. We have no court, no jail, and no fines. You do this out of respect for Lakota ways and what the spirits have told Elmer. If you cannot respect these ways, then please do everyone a favor (including yourself) and pray somewhere else.

People who have had a vision from the Thunder Beings, or the Spirits of the West, may have to honor the *heyokas*, as they are properly called. This might mean doing everything opposite from how others do things. Some people, especially men, may have the spirit of the opposite sex trapped inside of them. These people, *winktes*, may dress and act as a woman and would not be considered offensive in their behavior to men or women. Transvestites and homosexuals are not treated quite as nicely in most of American society, but in Lakota traditions, these people are considered sacred and have a role to play in the tribe.

As stated previously, Elmer Running has been a sundance leader for over twenty years. He has had a vision, which can only be delivered while a person is awake—and is delivered by the Lakota ancestors—when working with the sacred pipe, or *canunpa*. He is an interpreter who is in constant contact with the ancestors, animal spirits, and spirits from other places. Over the years, numerous spirits have communicated with Elmer to outline how he is to conduct ceremonies, how sun dancers should perform the rituals of the sun dance, how supporters should act and behave, and how visitors should be while near the sun-dance arbor. With these concepts in mind, here are some things that people might like to know to lead to good understanding of these ways.

A sun dancer is generally a person who carries a *canunpa*. Others may be giving thanks for some great thing the spirits have done or praying for loved ones who are in great need. Still others may have had a dream, interpreted by a medicine man or an interpreter, in which they support the sun dance by dancing. This *canunpa* was gifted to the individual by the spirits to help others to pray and help others be healthy. The *canunpa* will help provide and protect the pipe carrier, but it is a direct link to the spirits and the creator (Taku Skanskan, which literally means "mover of all things") to answer the prayers of others.

The sun dance is the most important of the seven sacred ceremonies of the Lakota Sioux Nation given to the people by the White Buffalo Calf Woman. Traditionally, the pipe is made by a carrier after a dream (which we have when we are asleep) or a vision (when one or more spirits come to you and speak to you in Lakota when you are awake, which has much greater significance than dreams), that is then interpreted by a medicine man or interpreter. The pipe can also be gifted by another sun dancer, family member, or friend. The pipe might also come to someone through a ceremony, such as being given the pipe that is tied onto the sundance tree. The pipe is honored in certain ways at all times, and this document is not meant to train someone on how to be a pipe carrier. Rarely does someone "buy" or "trade" to receive his or her pipe. If one is meant to be a pipe carrier, the spirits will make sure the individual receives a pipe in a good way. Few non-Indians receive a *canunpa* from the spirits.

When a sun dancer has a yearning or calling to dance, he or she commits to an altar. That altar has been given to a medicine man or interpreter in a vision. A sun dancer commits to a four-year cycle, honoring the four directions. Once the cycle is completed, it starts over again, but still at the same altar. No matter where the medicine man or interpreter holds the sun dance, the sun dancer is committed to be there. If for some reason (a very important one), the sun dancer cannot be there, he must ask the medicine man or interpreter to hold a special ceremony for them to honor their commitment. Elmer says the pipe never ends. That means that you dance until you die—and even then, it continues in the next life. If people miss a year of sun dancing, they give up a year of life later, according to what the spirits have told Elmer.

When an interpreter passes on, or the altar is taken away from the spirits, or he gives it back to the spirits, then the sun dancers can go to another altar. Many sun dancers came to the three altars that Elmer has been given under the direction of Martin High Bear right before he passed on to the next life. This is how it is done in a good way. Now these dancers follow the ways of the spirits who guide Elmer.

Therefore, only when the medicine man or interpreter returns the altar to the spirits, by death, by request, or by choice, should sun dancers decide to go to another altar. Dancers may leave an altar for personal reasons or if instructed in dreams by the spirits, but this should not happen often. In any case, people should dance at only one sun dance each year. The spirits have told Elmer that the sun dance will get tougher and people will have to be more traditional in supporting the pipe.

People do not pay to sun dance, to support, or to observe. People do donate things to help the sun-dance leader, the singers, and the sun dance. Since a medicine man or interpreter cannot charge to do ceremony, people donate food, clothing, transportation, and money to help him meet his day-to-day expenses, as he has no ordinary income. The singers may have jobs, but they commit to four days, and they pay for all their expenses. Donations to them are very helpful and appreciated by the singers, who many times have given up jobs to be at the sun dance. Food for the camp, firewood, rocks, and shelters for those who are less fortunate are always appreciated. Also, sun dancers who have completed their four-year cycle do a giveaway after the sun dance has finished. This may be any mixture of things—from clothing to books, to food, to ceremonial items, to gifts for the children and the elderly.

Sun dancers do not drink alcohol, do drugs of any kind, treat sex casually (they are monogamous), or speak badly of others. They follow this one path as a complete way of life. They gen-

erally do not practice another faith or religion, and they do not
participate in ceremonies that are contradictory to the way of
the sacred pipe as given to the Lakota people by White Buffalo
Calf Woman. This may include peyote ceremonies, mixed sweat
lodges (men and women should never sweat together), or ceremonies where the pipe is dishonored. That is hard to do all the time,
but as pipe carriers, they can be called on by people twenty-four
hours a day, seven days a week to pray with the *canunpa* the
spirits have given them. In that, there is no such thing as a "personal pipe." The pipe was a gift to the "people."

Those who cannot honor the pipe or honor their commitment
as a sun dancer must give the pipe back to the spirits or accept
the consequences of not doing so. The same is true of using alcohol and drugs. The spirits and Wakan Takan are not fooled, even
if humans are. Participants must accept the consequences of their
actions. If they leave an altar, they should leave the pipes they
used at that altar to the spirits or the sun-dance leader. The spirits
will provide a new one for their new altar, if they are meant to be
pipe carriers.

The sun dance has four components. Preparation is four days
and includes getting the sun-dance skirts and dresses ready, as
well as preparing for sun dance. People now generally do this all
year long, including purifying monthly and making prayer ties,
because they work and live far away. Four days are spent helping
to set up the sun-dance arbor and grounds and "purify" with
evening sweats each day. All sun dancers should be at purification for all four days, but that is hard in these modern times. The
last day of this purification is tree day, when the interpreter picks
a young boy and young girl who are virgins to ceremonially cut
down the sun-dance tree with the assistance of sun-dance helpers, who are picked by the sun-dance leader.

The four days of the sun dance are now typically held from
Thursday to Sunday. The final four days are known as *wopila*,

when sun dancers give thanks for their prayers being answered
and return to their homes. Many sun dancers also pray by
themselves once a year. This is known as *hanblecheyapi*. The
direct translation is "vision quest," though few ever receive a true
vision and usually not until someone is age fifty or beyond. If a
person is given a vision by the spirits, this is a time that it will
happen. Normally, one day and night are sufficient for this prayer
time. Sometimes, people will have a dream (which should be
interpreted by an interpreter or medicine man) wherein they are
required to stay longer, but rarely, if ever, should people go up
for longer than one day and one night. Rarely are people required
to suffer "on the hill" for four days and nights, but it does happen if that is what the spirits direct. Again, this is almost always
in a dream or in a vision (when one is awake and sober) interpreted by a medicine man or interpreter. Very few people ever
have true visions, and even then, they would probably have to be
fluent in Lakota and be able to understand ancient and spiritual
Lakota, which the spirits who work with the *canunpa* speak.
Other Indians need to know the language of their ancestors. Few
non-Indians ever get a vision, and even then, they would certainly have to have fluency in a particular Indian tongue, and it
would be by the decision of the spirits and under their direction,
which would be told to them by Elmer in ceremony.

Elmer will accept a pipe from almost anyone who wants to
sun dance, regardless of race, age, or nationality. In recent years,
some have been asked not to sun dance at the All Nations Sun
Dance if they did not follow instructions given to them by the
spirits (through Elmer or his designate), for mixing religions (not
following the Lakota path), for blaspheming the pipe or White
Buffalo Calf Woman, or for changing from altar to altar at whim.
Some people have charged money for people to pray with the
pipe that has been entrusted to them by the spirits. This is never

proper. The pipes belong to the spirits, and people should not charge for prayer.

For people who want to pierce, they must have their ropes on the tree when it goes up on Wednesday, or use someone else's. Sun dancers pierce only once a year. They need only pierce once on their bodies, although many pierce in two places on either the front or back. Rarely should anyone pierce in both the front and back in the same year. Generally, they pierce while tied to the tree, and rarely would someone need to pierce another way. Dragging buffalo skulls was an ancient sign of repentance, done in private and for some horrid offense, such as theft, rape, or murder. Sometimes, they may be dragged when all else has failed to save someone's life. Even then, it happened outside of the arbor.

Many people forget to have Elmer perform a *lowampi* ceremony to have the spirits doctor someone before they try to pray on their own during the sun dance through piercing. It was generally not used for prayer during the sun dance, and Elmer states that in the old days, maybe only one in ten sun dancers would pierce. Horses were not used, either, as these were introduced by the Europeans after they invaded North America and certainly could not have been used in ancient sun dances.

During the sun dance, alcohol, drugs, firearms, or other weapons, along with hate, jealousy, and bad feelings are left at the gate coming into the sun-dance grounds. Women wear skirts while in ceremonies or around ceremonies to show respect to White Buffalo Calf Woman. If they are having menstruation, or are on their moon time, they are very spiritual and can actually "drown out" the power of the pipe to transmit the people's prayers. So, out of respect to the needs of people who must use the pipe to pray, they stay away from areas where *canunpas* are loaded and ready to transmit the people's prayers.

Sun dancers wear sage wrist cuffs so they can be directed by other sun dancers and not be touched, as well as sage anklets and a crown of sage, which traditionally is held together by sinew. This keeps their thoughts and bodies pure after purification each morning. They may be covered by red cloth in strips or completely covered in cloth to honor one or more of the directions. Men wear cloth skirts of red or of colors honoring the four directions, Mother Earth, the *heyokas*, or the spirits of the sky. Women wear dresses with shawls around the waist, and each of the directions is honored by at least one woman, required for certain parts of the ceremony. Sun dancers' skirts should be simple and should only be the colors of the four directions, the earth, and the sky. Red for men is the traditional color. It may have ribbons of white, yellow, blue, green, black, and white to honor the directions.

Sun dancers commit to four full days of sun dancing. If dancers are unable to do this, then they should consider if they are really meant to sun dance. People have been fired from jobs to make their sun-dance commitment, as well as using their entire savings to get to the sun dance. That is out of respect, commitment, and honor. People who have serious physical handicaps are considered to be sun dancers, even if they cannot dance every round. They remain under the shade portion of the arbor, praying while the other dancers continue with the ceremony. No sun dancer should leave the arbor or the *inipi* lodge area during the sun dance each day. Fire keepers or security people can get things they need, excluding drink, food, cigarettes, salves (Bengay, etc.), or other things that will make the sun dance easier.

Sun dancers bring only a blanket to the sun-dance arbor. That is the only comfort that they get. They must not touch each other, and joking and idle talk are really inappropriate for sun dancers, who have committed four days to pray for the people, including loved ones, friends, and even enemies. If people cannot do this for this time period, then perhaps they are not yet ready in their lives to sun dance. Sun dancers try not to lie down or sleep during the breaks, as they are meant to pray. Sage, cedar, and sweet grass are appropriate for cuts, sores, and piercings.

Dancers attached to the tree for four days traditionally take no food or fluids for the entire time they sun dance. They leave only to relieve themselves. They have nothing but a mat of sage to protect them, as the tree takes care of their needs during the four days. Some may be attached for a shorter period, but generally they request to stay on for four days. Otherwise, they can just pierce during a piercing round. Many people pierce for the wrong reason, and they should remember that the proper way to do healing ceremonies is to put up a *lowampi* or *yuwipi* ceremony in a good way.

Flesh offerings can be given by anyone but must be taken by a sun dancer. These may be done in groups of one, four, or seven (although seven is rare). One flesh offering a year is sufficient for any person, according to what the spirits have told Elmer.

In honor of the White Buffalo Calf Woman, who delivered the pipe to the people, men treat women with respect, honor, and dignity, and women wear skirts or dresses, which cannot be seen through when they get wet or show a woman's private parts when she sits or bends over. Men should not look at a woman in anything but a respectful way. Married individuals should not be alone with others of the opposite sex, married or unmarried. Men traditionally turn their backs when the women enter or leave the *inipi* lodge to give them privacy and dignity.

People should not be getting into heated arguments or fight during purification and the sun dance and are considered part of the family or tribe while on the sun-dance grounds.

Sun dancers do not advertise their status as sun dancers. They do not show their scars in public and should have their bodies covered outside of the sun dance. Men do so by covering their chests and backs, women and men by covering their upper arms.

When in and around the arbor, people should not wear shiny or reflective materials. This includes jewelry, watches, earrings, eyeglasses, or shiny materials like sequins. Sun dancers do wear medicine bags, but not crystals or rocks that are shiny. Sun dancers should not have any clothing with reflective material (such as shiny threads). Men and women wear their hair straight, with no braids or ties. People should not wear shoes when they are in the arbor, while the tree is up. This is not true for *heyokas*, though, who have to follow their vision. They do many things differently, and they follow directions that are often private and known only to them and the interpreter. It is not for others to judge anyone in the arbor, as sun dancers believe that the arbor is *wakan* (sacred) and that it is almost impossible to do anything wrong under the strict guidance of the spirits and the interpreter. They will let the sun dancers know if something is being done in a bad way, usually through Elmer or by some action. People also do not assume they know why something happens in the arbor. Only the spirits, the creator, and White Buffalo Calf Woman know, and sometimes they will tell Elmer, and he can tell people why a thing happened. Often, something is private, and the sun dancers and supporters may not ever know what the interpreter has told someone about an incident. So we try not to assume or be judgmental of others. Elmer says we have no right to push anyone away from the sacred circle. The spirits protect the pipes and the arbor. If someone is in the arbor and if someone is there year in and year out, then they are where they are supposed to be. It is not up to people to gossip or say if and how things should be. Only Elmer has the right to do this as the sun-dance leader, and he will tell certain people to tell people what the spirits say. So listen to people when they say, "Elmer told me to tell you this," as rarely will he talk directly to someone about something done in a bad way. That is the role of other sun dancers.

If you want to dance to help support the dancers, feel free to spread a blanket or towel to dance on. Dancers do not wear any makeup, sun blocks, ointments, or salves to protect them from the earth, the sun, or the other elements. They have faith in Wakan Takan, the creator, and the spirits that gave the vision to Elmer Running. The tree protects them. If they are sick, hungry, or thirsty, you will see them go and pray to the tree for help. It can give the dancers everything they need to complete the sun dance.

Sun dancers carry fans of sacred bird feathers or plumes, sage, and their pipes when they enter and leave the arbor every day. Others should never look at, speak to, or interact with sun dancers during the ceremony. This begins with the morning purification and ends after the evening purification. Only sun dancers can enter the rest area, where the dancers stay during breaks. Sun dancers cannot eat, drink, or smoke during the ceremony each day. Many fast all four days, so please be considerate of them. If they stay in or near the arbor, please observe their need for prayer and only approach them if they ask for assistance.

If you have prayer ties, flesh offerings, or flags that you wish to have attached to the tree, a sun dancer may put them on if they have purified for that day. Only sun dancers touch the tree at any time before it is felled, during the ceremony, or after the ceremony, unless given permission by the sun-dance leader, Elmer Running, or by one of his helpers after they have asked his permission.

All people coming into the arbor to support dancers' piercing, during naming ceremonies, or to pledge for next year's sun dance must purify in a sweat lodge before entering the arbor. There are no exceptions to this very important procedure. People are escorted in by the south gate if praying or supporting or at the north gate if pledging to sun dance. Please put sage in your right hand, and the escort will grab this to lead you to your spot. Never touch sun dancers with your hands. If you want to support a sun-dancer piercing, obey the commands of the other sun dancers first. You can touch the sun dancer with sage, one of our most sacred and healing herbs. When sun dancers break, they are not to be touched by others unless so directed by the sun-dance leader. A sun dancer will lead the person who has successfully broken from the tree to each of the four directions, which they and only they honor by turning to the four directions. The sun dancer will then be brought to the tree to give thanks and pray for his brother the tree, who is passing on to the next life. The sun dancer will then be brought back to his or her place in the perfect circle, and he or she then honors the four directions. Sun dancers and supporters do not need to honor the four directions at each gate. They do so only when they return to their spots in the perfect circle.

Sun dancers purify by themselves each day before and after they enter the arbor during the sun dance. No one should sweat with them at those times. If people want to sweat, they can sweat with a sun dancer in a seven-rock, one-round sweat during the breaks.

Pets are forbidden, and children should not disrupt the ceremony or the camp. If they cannot be properly supervised or controlled, do not think of the sun dance as a personal day-care center. It is not. Automobiles should also be kept away from the arbor, as there are many reflective materials on them that distract the spirits. Please honor everyone's personal belongings.

One must never cross the east gate, as this is where the spirits and sun dancers enter. Even *heyokas* are very respectful of this. People can enter the arbor from the north or south gates. At the end of each round, the sun-dance leader will choose a person to receive the pipe and a sun dancer who will offer the pipe. If you are asked to receive the pipe, proceed to the south gate. Rub your hands with sage, hold your hands palm up with sage in them, and take the pipe to the fourth offering. After you are done smoking it with friends, family, or others, return to the south gate and await the person who gave the pipe to you. They will take it back.

Above all, respect the Mother Earth by treating her as your good friend. Do not litter, throw trash on her, needlessly abuse her, cut down plants and trees without asking permission and offering tobacco and before making your best efforts to save a tree or plant from needless destruction. There is lots of firewood that is already there for the taking without cutting down trees that are alive and well.

A lot has been said about who can pour a sweat. The Stone People's Lodge is one of the seven sacred ceremonies given to the Lakota Sioux people by White Buffalo Calf Woman. As practiced by the Lakota Sioux, the spirits have told Elmer Running that only a person who is a pipe carrier and knows how the ritual should be performed (including the appropriate songs in Lakota, how the fire is set up, how the altar is set up, how the lodge is built, and all the details that make the ceremony) and either a sun dancer or a person who has done his or her annual *hanblecheyapi* and is not charging money for the ceremony should run a sweat lodge. This should be done only by having a person come to the pipe carrier and offering tobacco to the spirits and asking for help from the spirits and God. A woman on her moon time might ask another to do so. Also, the lodge must have been blessed by Elmer, and the prayer ties should be done before the ceremony. In Lakota ceremonies, men and women do not perform this ceremony together. There are obvious sexual problems that can arise, but there are other spiritual reasons. If men and woman are to share ceremony, men sweat first, do not sing the spirit leaving song, the women sweat, and they do not need to sing the spirit invitation song, but they then sing a song giving thanks to the spirits for coming and hearing and hopefully helping to answer the people's prayers. Elmer has said the spirits are emphatic about this, regardless of what he or others may think as individual humans.

Before, during, and after sun dance, Elmer's wife, Patti, can be of great help in telling people what they need to do to prepare for the sun dance as a dancer, supporter, or visitor. Please remember that they open their house to everyone 361 days a year, that they work long hours with no expectation of reward or thanks, and they have limited income. The house is off-limits during purification and the sun dance to anyone without the Runnings' explicit permission. Please be considerate and help with household chores and with setting up the sun-dance grounds, the ceremony house, the Stone People's lodges, and the surrounding area. Please remember that the neighbors that you upset and see only four to eight days each year live next to Elmer and Patti all year long. Be polite when in the local area, be respectful of the area in general, and be a welcome guest. This is a good time to remember that great Lakota rule: Do unto others as you would have them do unto you.

When you begin this sacred ritual, remember me as you fill the pipe: Do this, and whatever you desire will come true.